The Erg Book:

375+ of the Greatest Indoor Rowing Workouts of All Time

The Short and Snarky Coxswains

& Peter Cannia

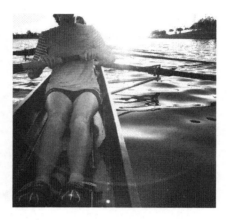

This book is dedicated to Cindy Craver,
whom we have to think is looking down on us
from the stroke seat of an eight
on a ridiculously flat piece
of water somewhere.

We miss you, Cindy.

TABLE OF CONTENTS

ACKNOWLEDGEMENTS

Thank you to our fellow coaches, program staff, family and friends, but mostly to our rowers, who unwittingly tested these workouts and saved our readers from the truly bad ones. We'd like to thank our TTLR masters and TJC juniors who braved the never-ending season of winter training that stretched until May, Lance Matheson, Denise Lee and John Ciani for continuing their international modeling careers on these very pages, editor Diane Ingalsbe, book designer Janet Mrazek, Alicia Jerger and Ryan Allison for making it all possible and especially the folks at Bridgestone for giving us the rare opportunity to turn lemons into lemonade. We'd also like to say thanks to all of our Short and Snarky readers, followers and podcast listeners. Without you guys this book would never have happened.

ABOUT THIS BOOK

There are many measures of what makes a truly great rower, indoor or otherwise. World Records. Hardware. Membership in the 20 million meter club. Suffice to say we are not truly great indoor rowers. We've never won C.R.A.S.H.-B.s, we didn't row on a National Team, and we sure never went to the Olympics, except to watch from the back of the stadium. If you are looking for guidance from a world-class rower, you might want to consider another book. There are plenty of options out there.

This book is written for people like the ones we see every day on our high school and masters rowing teams and at the gym – people like us. The ones who knock around dilapidated boathouses in the hinterlands, toiling in obscurity during the off-season when the water is frozen. The ones who row on the one crummy erg in the corner of the gym or at home alone in their basement, never sure if they're really doing it right. The fitness training class warriors who boast of splits that cause 'real' rowers to snicker. You know who you are, and this book is for you. We will help you make your boathouse, garage or rec center a happier place, give you ideas to quell the erg boredom and provide a glimmer of fun in the dark days of winter training.

ABOUT THE SHORT AND SNARKY COXSWAINS

The Short and Snarky Coxswains have turned themselves into a very minor Internet rowing phenomenon over the past few years, bringing wit and humor to the sometimes-staid world of rowing. Occasionally real journalists write them up, but most of the time they just make people laugh on social media and in their occasional iTunes "Way Nuff Rowing Podcast." What's more, they are real rowers, coxswains and rowing coaches.

Their first book, *The Short and Snarky Guide to Coxing and Rowing*, available on Amazon, has been lauded across the rowing community for its humor and insight into rowing on actual water. While it hasn't yet made the *New York Times* bestseller list, it has sold more copies than they could possibly have expected in their wildest dreams.

One of the Short and Snarky Coxswains spent her collegiate rowing career getting tossed into rivers and ponds up and down the East Coast and can't figure out exactly when that weird rash developed. A Head of the Charles medalist, Badger State Games three-sport champion (a competition for residents of one of America's least fit states) and winner of the 'best stake boat holder on the lake' every time she touches a hull, her vagabond lifestyle and sparkling personality have taken her through 11 different rowing clubs in eight U.S. states. In two decades of coaching, she has picked up the US Rowing Level III coaching certification and has sat through the CPR/First Aid class at least 20 times, an all-time Red Cross record. She currently coaches a masters rowing team in Arizona where she occasionally spies road-runners from the coaching launch and is ready to spring into action if someone chokes on a large bite of steak during practice.

The other Short and Snarky Coxswain started rowing in her middle school years, and after her high school team's heyday – where she and her crews rowed themselves to greatness in numerous juniors events – she moved on to coaching for a high school club team. The brains behind the Short and Snarky Rowing social media presence and podcast, she is a US Rowing Masters Nationals champion, marketing superstar and all around jokester and teller of bad puns. Voted four-time 'most likely to hit a fishing boat while rowing at full speed,' although she only stands five feet tall, don't get between her and an all-you-can-eat baked potato bar. She coxes, coaches and rows in the southwestern desert of Tempe, Arizona.

Short and Snarky Rowing can be found at @shortandsnarkyrowing and @shortandsnarky on just about all the social media sites you can think of. Email us at shortandsnarkyrowing@gmail.com.

ABOUT PETER CANNIA

Pete has coached crew in California and Arizona for the better part of two decades. Pete started coaching because he took a vow of poverty, and his life lacked the aggravation and mental abuse that you can only find by coaching. Along with rowing medals, 80s band groupies and 'best hair' awards, Pete specializes in racking up athletic training and fitness credentials. He has a degree in exercise and wellness, holds the US Rowing Level III coaching certification and is a Certified Strength and Conditioning Specialist (CSCS), a Certified Personal Trainer (NSCA-CPT), a USAW Sports Performance Weightlifting Coach and a CrossFit Level I Trainer. He currently coaches high school and masters rowers in Tempe, Arizona, where he cruises the lake picking up discarded malt liquor bottles and imploring rowers to 'stop killing fish!' with their oars.

INTRODUCTION

Love and Hate on the Erg

Ergs. Ergometers. Ergos. Rowing machines. Indoor rowers. Whatever you call them, most rowers, whether they row on the water or on land, have a complex relationship with the machine itself. On one hand, you have to appreciate anything that can provide you with such a second-by-second glimpse into your physical output. Stories of triumph on the erg are legendary – the woman who lost 200 pounds erging, the girl who qualified for a collegiate scholarship in rowing despite never pulling an oar through the water or that guy in England who passed the time during a prison sentence setting world erg records. The erg truly can change your life.

On the other hand, there is the reality of erging. Sometimes ergs send you running for the nearest trash can, give you the 'erg lung' death cough or make you crawl into a fetal position on a dirty concrete floor. The erg can make a grown man cry and make experienced rowers throw up their hands in exasperation as though it was the first time they'd ever sat on an erg seat. The erg can break you down mentally like nothing else. We've been there, and we get it. This book is full of workouts and advice to make your workouts better. However, we're not going to lie and tell you it will all be butterflies and rainbows. If you're doing it right, sometimes it is going to be hard, and sometimes it is going to hurt. Consider yourself warned, and check with your doctor before diving in head first into the amazing world of indoor rowing.

Safety First

The erg can be a great tool to get into shape, rehab from an injury or just stay active as you age (just ask one of the octogenarians at any indoor erg race). However, anyone who isn't already physically fit should only proceed on the advice of their physician, and new rowers are advised to go slow. We include introductory workouts for this very reason. Making sure to set the damper on an easier setting and not overdoing it are key when you are starting out, especially if you have limited capabilities or are not in great shape currently.

ALL ABOUT THE ERG

Erg technology is pretty simple. You pull on the handle of the erg, which drives a flywheel, which generates power, which is quantified on a screen. Each manufacturer's erg models are slightly different, but all rely on the same basic premise – pull hard on the erg and generate numbers on the screen. While there are a number of manufacturers, including WaterRower, Stamina, Kettler and ProRower, ergs manufactured by Concept2 are the original, most popular and widely-used worldwide. With new models coming out periodically, most rowing clubs and gyms will likely have a diversity of models.

Parts of the Erg

If you're new to the erg, do your best to familiarize yourself with the basic parts. As we mentioned above, each manufacturer will have a slightly different erg layout and parts, so adapt to fit your preferred model. Here are some of the key parts of the machine we all love to hate:

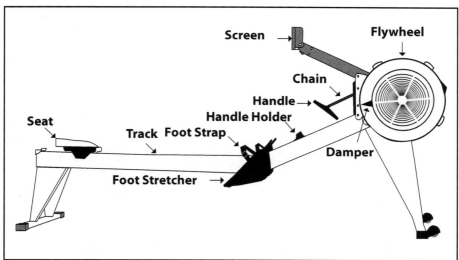

Erg Screens and What They Mean

Screens are slightly different among the models and among the manufacturers, but all will share similar data, just in slightly different configurations. Don't be afraid of the numbers on the erg screen. While erg screens display other useful information such as watts, calories, and projected splits, the four major numbers, discussed in the next section, are the primary focus when you're erging.

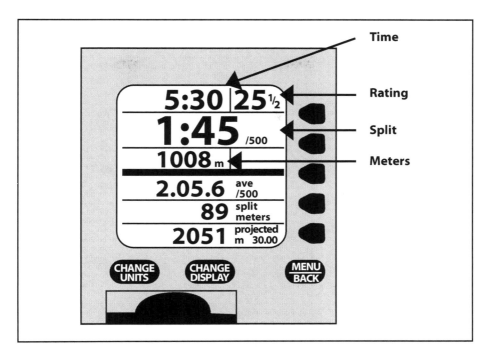

Don't be afraid of the numbers on the erg screen. While erg screens display other useful information such as watts, calories, and projected splits, the four major numbers, discussed below, are the primary focus when you're erging.

When you first come face to face with an erg screen, all of the numbers can be daunting. We're here to walk you through it. The four major numbers on any erg screen will be rating, time, split and meters. While ergs have other settings (watts, calories, etc.), the four major numbers are the primary focus while you're erging.

Meters. Ergs measure distance rowed in meters. Ergs can be set to show either meters that the rower has already pulled or meters left to pull in the workout. Meters are abbreviated as 'm,' as in '500m.'

Rating. Rating is the average number of strokes pulled in 60 seconds. This is also known as 'strokes per minute,' 'stroke rate,' 'stroke rating' or 'rate.' Generally this number will be between 14 and 42. For example, if the number reads 24, that means at the pace you're currently rowing you would pull an average of 24 strokes in a minute. In this book we abbreviate rating as 'SPM' (strokes per minute).

Time. Erg timers can be set to show either elapsed time or time remaining in the workout. This is typically easy to spot because it looks like a stopwatch. Numbers will read in minutes and seconds; for example, 02:34 or 27:16.

Split. Your split is the amount of time (in minutes and seconds) it will take you to pull 500m on the erg. For example, a 2:05 on your screen would equate to your taking two minutes and five seconds to complete a 500m piece, if you continue pulling at the same pressure. Splits can range from upwards of 6:00 when the fly wheel is barely moving to less than 1:20 when pulled at max pressure by an elite athlete. Rowers often ask what a "good" split should be. While this differs for every person based on age, fitness level and weight, most indoor rowers will see splits somewhere between 1:35 and 2:45 on a typical piece.

Programming Your Workout

The last thing we'll say about erg screens is that you want to spend a little time figuring out how to program in your workouts. Most newer model ergs have pre-programmed workouts already in them, but they can also be set to things like 'just row,' 'set distance' and 'set time.' It is well worth the hassle of figuring this out, either by tracking down the user's manual online or by trial and error. You'll also want to figure out how to recall data using the 'history' or 'recall' function.

We also highly recommend that you visit Concept2's website (or those for other manufacturers) for more information on using, programming, maintaining and storing your erg.

ADJUSTING THE ERG TO FIT YOUR BODY

We've been coaching rowing for a while now, and you would be shocked at the differences from one person's body to the next person's body. We're not talking about height or weight (although those are things to consider); we're talking about proportion and ratio, length of torso, legs, feet, general flexibility and reach. It is essential that you make the erg fit your own body. Here are a few ways to adjust your erg:

Damper Setting

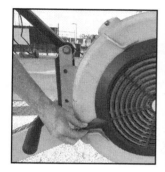 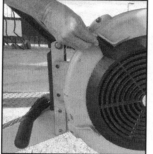 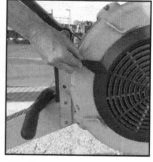

Low number setting closes damper, restricting airflow into the flywheel and making it easier to spin, which is particularly useful during long, steady-state pieces.

High number setting opens damper, letting air into the flywheel and making it harder to spin, which is particularly useful during shorter, TR type workouts.

Moderate number setting lets some air into the flywheel, which is a good all-purpose setting for most workouts.

You may notice a dial on your erg that makes it easier or harder to pull on the handle. This is known as the damper. Generally changing the erg damper increases or decreases the amount of airflow against the erg's flywheel, and accordingly makes it easier or more difficult to pull the chain or handle. A word to the wise – unless you are rowing at the most elite levels, are on a competitive rowing team under a coach's supervision or have years of indoor rowing experience, give your back a break and keep the damper setting low. On Concept2 ergs, this means no higher than a 3 or 4 (out of 10) setting. There are too many horror stories about people setting dampers on the highest level and then doing a bunch of short pieces, only to collapse and die from cardiac arrest. Family members of deceased rowers also have a tendency to sue coaches, trainers and gyms for these types of accidents, so don't say we didn't warn you.

Foot Stretchers

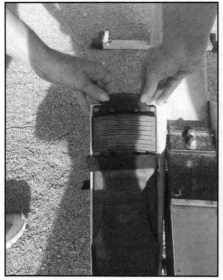
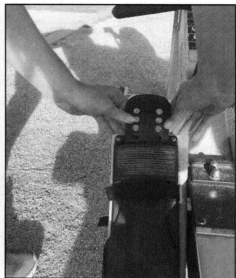

Foot stretchers in lowest position　　　　*Foot stretchers in highest position*

The foot stretchers on an erg are adjustable, and you should adjust them according to the length of your lower legs and your overall flexibility. Generally speaking, if you have long legs, you'll want to drop the foot stretchers down close to the floor. On Concept2 ergs, this will make all of the holes in the foot stretchers disappear below the main foot plate. If you have really short legs and small feet, you'll want to lift up the foot stretchers away from the floor. On Concept2 ergs, this will mean lots of the holes on the foot stretchers are showing.

Here are a few more variables:

- Long legs overall, but short shin bones – adjust the foot stretchers higher than you would if your legs were proportional.

- Shorter legs, but have really flexible hamstrings and Achilles tendons – keep the foot stretchers lower than you would for someone with less flexibility and short legs.

- Low flexibility in hamstrings and Achilles tendons – set the foot stretchers higher than you would for someone with your leg length.

- Big feet, we mean big feet, like size 13 or larger, you'll want to drop the foot stretchers lower than you otherwise would for someone of your height.

Seat Pads

Like length of legs, many people have disproportionately short tor-sos. You'll probably never realize just how disproportionate you are until you start rowing, but here is a clue – if you often feel short when you sit down, relative to other people of the same height, you might be a contender for a short torso award. If you have this lucky ana-tomical feature, get yourself a seat pad. Seat pads come in all shapes and sizes. You can make your own for pennies out of foam from a home improvement store, or you can pay a ton for a fancy gel-based one designed for rowing. We recommend starting out with the cheap foam option and adding or subtracting based on how it goes. De-pending on your quirky anatomy, you might only need a centimeter of padding, or you might need to get yourself a few of those foam knee pads made for gardening, cut to fit the seat, and duct tape the pieces together. If you have a bony rear, you might also be a great candidate for a seat pad, but don't go overboard on the padding if you have a long torso, or you will create other problems for yourself.

BASIC ROWING TECHNIQUE

The Basic Rowing Stroke

The stroke has two basic parts, the drive and the recovery.

THE DRIVE

The drive is the part of the stroke where you are generating power and exerting effort. The drive begins at the catch, continues as you push your legs down, swing your back open and pull your arms in and ends at the release. If you were rowing on real water, the release would be the point where the blades exit the water.

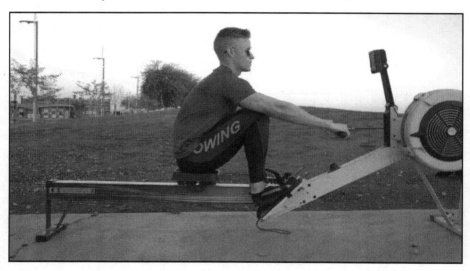

The catch. The catch is where you begin your stroke. Your body should be at full compression. This means that the shins should be straight up and down, perpendicular to the floor. Heels should be off the footplate, and you should be on the balls of your feet. The back is straight with a lean forward, with a slight arch of the lower back; shoulders should be up and relaxed. The arms should be fully extended, not dropped down on the knees or broken at the elbows, and wrists should be flat. Hands should be relaxed. There is a natural tendency in lower skill level rowers to dive forward at the catch. Remember to keep your hands up at the catch, head and chin up and eyes forward.

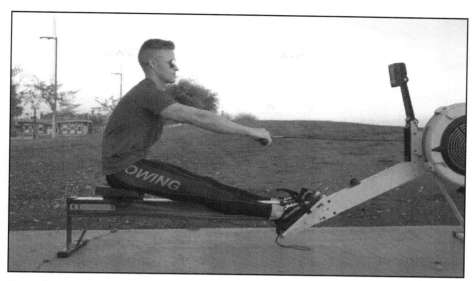

Leg drive. The leg drive portion begins as legs are pressed down. Remember to connect your feet with the foot stretchers, moving from pushing off the balls of the feet to pushing your heels down to the plate. The body should remain in a forward leaning position, and arms should remain straight.

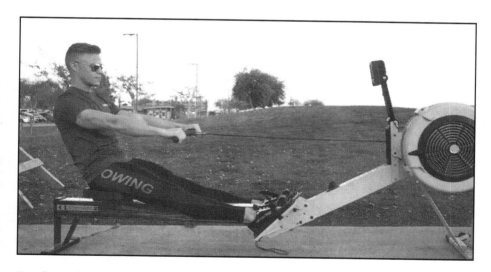

Back swing. As you are more than halfway through with the leg drive, you should begin to start to open up your back. Arms should continue to be outstretched straight and forward, with shoulders tall and relaxed. As the seat moves to the back of the tracks, swing your back open toward the back end of the erg. This position is called the 'layback'. If done well, you will experience an almost Zen-like state called 'swing'. This rarely happens, so if you have yet to experience it, don't worry. Newer rowers have a tendency to open their backs up too early or yank with the back. During the drive, remember not to open up your back early. Instead, focus on pushing with the legs, adding the back as an "add on" to the legs. If done right, the bulk of the stroke is done primarily with the legs (60%+) while the back is secondary (~15-20%).

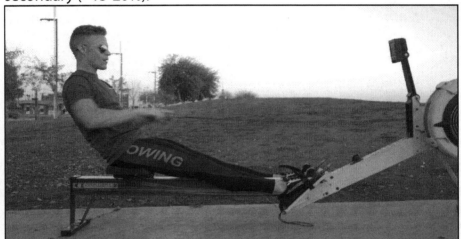

Arms in. The second to last part of the drive is the arms coming in. The arms should start to break at the elbows after you begin your layback. Elbows should be drawn at a comfortable position beyond the sides of the body, and the handle should continue toward your chest until just before the body. Remember to relax your shoulders, keep the wrists flat and maintain the connection between your feet and the foot stretchers. There is a natural tendency in newer rowers to break their wrists, drop the handle toward their laps or otherwise 'crank' on the handle in a downward motion. Remember to continue to pull the handle in toward the middle of your chest to your mark.

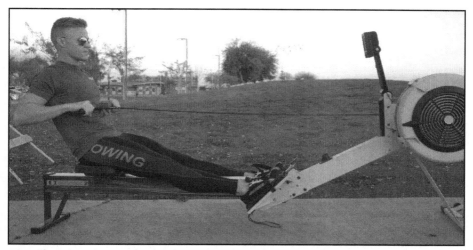

The finish. The end of the stroke is called 'the finish' or 'the release.' The backs of your thumbs should graze your shirt, but not slam into your body. At this point you should push your hands away from the body.

THE RECOVERY

The recovery is the part of the stroke where you are moving forward, back toward the erg screen, and preparing to take another catch. The recovery starts at the finish as you bring your hands away from your body. The recovery, like the drive, has three major parts and is basically the same as the drive, but done in reverse order.

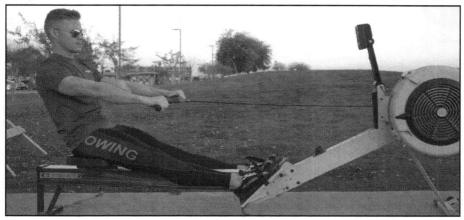

Arms away. At the finish you'll remain in the layback position as you push your arms away. A common problem in newer rowers is getting 'stuck' with the hands at the finish or stopping momentum at the finish. Instead, focus on pushing your hands away at the same speed you brought them into the body, without any stoppage or hitch.

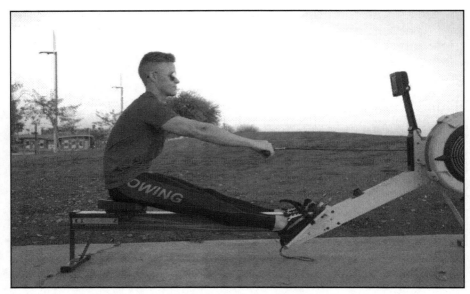

Body over. As soon as the hands come away, you'll want to swing your body forward from the hips. This is called 'body preparation'. You should maintain this body angle throughout the rest of the recovery.

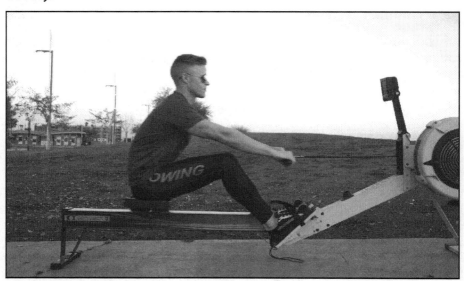

Legs up. As the body comes over, you will start to compress your legs forward, drawing nearer to the erg screen as you come up the slide. A common problem in newer rowers is rushing forward too quickly. Instead, focus on engaging the hamstrings and decelerating as you come forward.

Breaking the Stroke Down

When you're starting out with indoor rowing, whether it is your first time or just the beginning of a new workout, we highly recommend breaking down the erg stroke. Take it slow, and make sure you focus on good technique before worrying at all about power. You can start by taking some strokes with just your legs (no back or arms), then gradually add in the back and finally the arms, or rowing with arms only, then arms and body only and then legs only. Your warm up is a great opportunity to mix it up and take some time to review the basics.

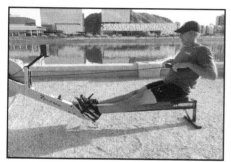 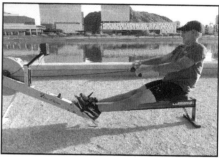

Arms Only Rowing. Row arms only, focusing on keeping the hands moving in a continuous loop. The legs stay completely flat and don't move, and the back stays in the layback position and does not move.

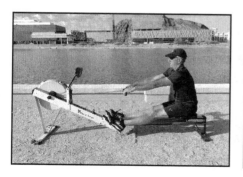 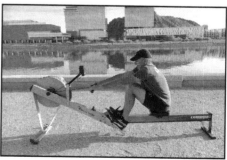

Legs Only Rowing. Legs only rowing involves moving up and down the track (bringing the handle along) using only the legs. The arms and back remain in the catch position, with the arms outstretched and flat, and the body pivoted forward off the hips.

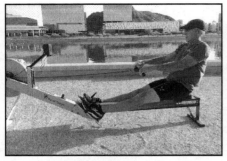 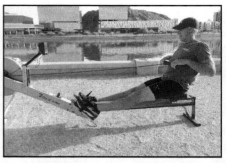

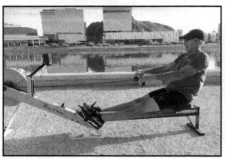 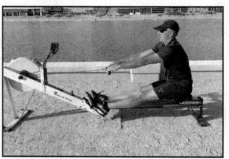

Arms and Body Only Rowing. This involves rowing with the arms and body only, focusing on pivoting forward and backward with the hips and moving the arms and hands in a continuous loop. The legs stay completely flat and do not move.

Setting Your Marks

Another great way to start your row off on the right note is to check your marks. This is an 'on the water' rowing term that can apply to ergs as well.

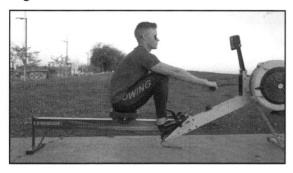

Mark the Catch. First, go to the catch position. Make sure you're sitting up, your shins are nice and straight up and down, you have your hands up, flat and even and have a nice arch in your lower back. Now, in that position, look at the level of your hands relative to the erg screen. That is the point you are aiming towards with your hands on each and every stroke. Many rowers like to mark that height with a piece of tape or sticker, so it's easy to aim towards.

Mark the Finish. Then go to the finish position with hands by the body. Again, make sure you're sitting up, the oar handle is pulled in at mid chest level, your elbows are relaxed and your wrists are flat. Mark that position

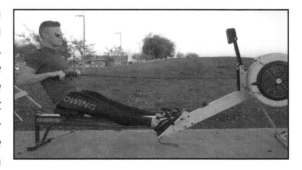

on your body by tapping the backs of the thumbs against your chest. Again, this is the height you're pulling towards on each and every stroke. Erging is pretty simple if you move the hands between point A (your mark at the catch) and point B (your mark at the finish).

Efficiency Curves

Yet another way to start off on the right foot with indoor rowing, and to see all of the technical problems with your rowing stroke, is to use the feature on your erg known as an efficiency curve or force curve. This is a visual depiction of your power during the stroke. Elite rowers will have force curves that look like a perfect parabola – a nice arch that peaks in the middle. Checking out your force curves from time to time provides valuable insights on technique flaws and where your power is coming from. Here are a few specific examples of force curves, both good and bad:

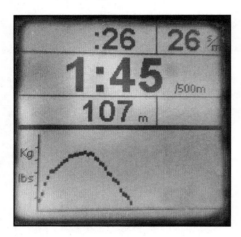

This is a good basic force curve. You can see how it makes a nice even arch.

A low, but consistently arched, curve suggests one thing – you're doing things right when it comes to transitions, but not generating much power. Low curves like the one in the picture are typical when you're first starting, on lower pressure pieces and during warm ups and cool downs.

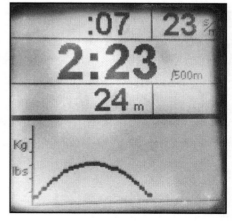

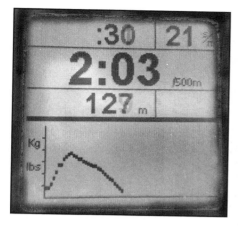

Here you can see what it looks like when you make a poor transition between the catch and the legs pushing down. Look at the big spike and the drop off. This isn't a terrible force curve, but the arch should be smoother. This suggests that the rower is loading too much on the back at the beginning and possibly pausing slightly after starting to open the back before driving the legs instead of pushing off the legs efficiently from the catch. If your force curve looks like this, focus on delaying opening the back and a smooth swing off the hips when you do start to open the back.

In this force curve, you can see generally weak power (see the low overall arch of the curve) and a poor transition from the catch to the main part of the drive, suggesting that the rower is opening up the back too early and putting too much load on the back as opposed to using the legs to push. If your force curve looks like this, concentrate on getting more power off of your legs by transitioning

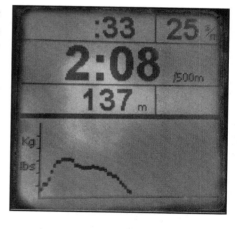

from weight on the balls of your foot at the catch to connecting your heels to the foot stretcher during the drive to generate efficient power, delaying opening the back and a smooth swing off the hips when you do start to open the back.

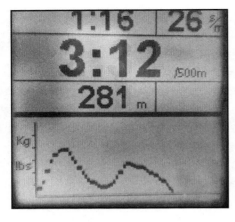

A force curve with two arches and a dip in between is indicative of bad transitions between the various parts of the stroke. Here in this example, the first arch suggests that the rower threw open the back too early (arch 1), dropped the power off during the leg drive and tried to crank the hands really hard at the finish (arch 2). This is a really inefficient stroke and a good way to hurt your back. If your force curves look like this, focus on delaying opening the back, doing most of the work with your legs and smoothly bringing your arms in.

A force curve that starts out really low and then barely arches up at the end suggests overall lack of power and an attempt by the rower to crank the back midway through or toward the end of the drive. This is likely a very short stroke with almost no power off of the feet. Overall this is a really inefficient stroke and could hurt your back. If your force curve looks like this, put your effort into getting in the right position at the catch with your shins nice and straight and sitting up tall.

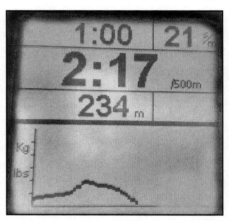

Then concentrate on getting more power off of your legs by transitioning from weight on the balls of your feet at the catch to connecting your heels to the foot stretcher during the drive to generate efficient power. At the end of the stroke, concentrate on smoothly bringing your arms in at the end (not 'cranking' them in).

The force curve doesn't lie. If your curves have some of these problems, you're likely falling victim to one or more of the common erg mistakes below. Keep the force curve screen up while you're doing your workouts, and consider adding a large mirror or camera, so you can see exactly what you're doing wrong.

COMMON ERG MISTAKES

Whether you've looked at your force curves or you're just starting out, there are a host of common erg mistakes that tend to trip up newer rowers. This is a short list of some of the most common mistakes new indoor rowers make. The more you can focus on starting off with good technique (and the muscle memory that comes with it) in your early rowing days, the more quickly your performance will improve and the less likely you will be to injure yourself. Here are a few common mistakes:

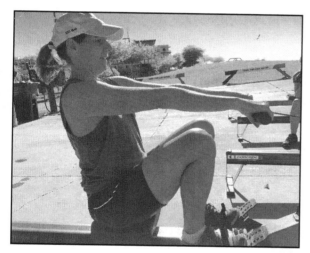

Opening the Back Up Too Early. This very common mistake happens when you throw open your back before driving your legs. This is a great way to injure your back and makes you row far less efficiently. Instead, focus on driving the legs first and then opening the back up.

Frog Legs. This mistake occurs when you open your knees up on either the drive or on the recovery. This mistake saps your power and throws the entire stroke off. Focus on keeping your knees closer together (within a few inches) and pushing off evenly on both feet.

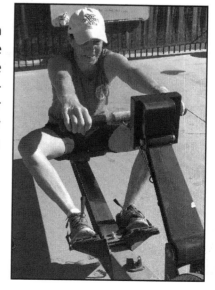

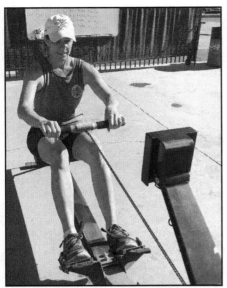

Arms Bent on Drive or Recovery. Rowing with your arms bent absolutely ruins any power and is just plain bad rowing. Focus on keeping your elbows straight throughout the entire stroke, except at the very end when you bring your hands to the body at the finish.

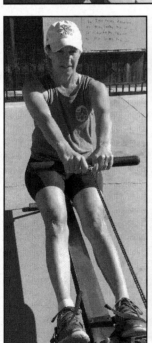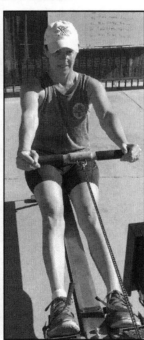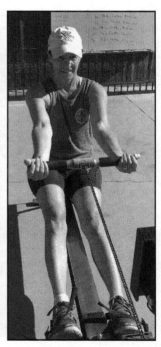

Poor Hand Position. We've seen rowers try all sorts of novel hand positions, including hands too close together, hands at the very ends of the handle and even hands upside down. You want to grip the handle right in the middle of the grip with hands shoulder width apart.

Pulling in Too High/Rowing Over a Barrel. Pulling in too high is a very common mistake. It is very difficult to maximize your power

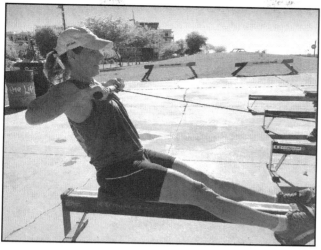

when your oar handle is coming dangerously close to your neck. A related problem is 'rowing over a barrel,' where the chain starts and ends at about the correct handle height, but in the middle of the drive, the rower exerts an upward lift on the chain before bringing it back to mid chest level. Focus on pulling the chain in a straight line to the body. For women we recommend pulling in to your 'mark' at the bottom of the sports bra line and for men at mid chest level.

Pulling in Too Low. The other end of the spectrum is pulling in too low, also known as 'dumping into the lap,' where a rower brings the

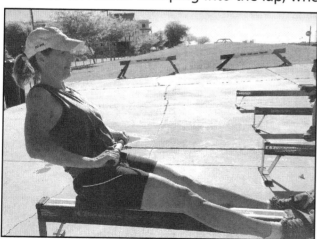

chain down on an angle toward his or her lap. Focus on pulling the chain in a straight line to the body. For women we recommend pulling in to your 'mark' at the bottom of the sports bra line and for men at mid chest level.

Diving at the Catch. Diving into the catch is a general term for the common problem of dropping either the head or the hands (or both) down at the catch position. If you find yourself looking at the floor, throwing your head back or grazing the handle on the base of the erg, these are all signs you're diving at the catch. At the catch you should be focusing on sitting up, arching the lower back and getting your chin up and eyes forward.

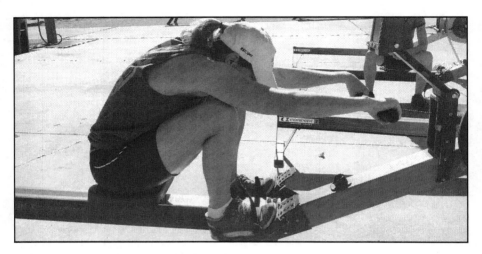

A. Incorrectly dropping the head.

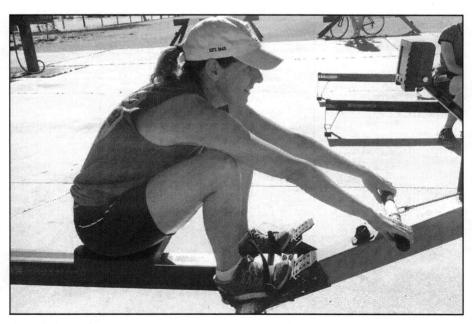

B. Incorrectly dropping the hands.

CALCULATING A BASELINE FOR WORKOUTS

All of the workouts in this book are based on splits (the average time it takes you to row 500m over a set, longer distance). In order to effectively do the workouts, you'll have to know your average split for a 2k test (2000 meters, as fast as you can go) and 6k test (6000 meters, as fast as you can go). When you're starting out, it might seem impossible to pull that many meters at full power in a single sitting. Other rowers may also have scared you about how much a 2k test hurts (They're right!). If that is the case, start slow with the introductory workouts in this book, and gradually work your way up to baseline testing. In our experience, 6k tests are slightly less mentally challenging and less painful, so as a beginner you might want to start with that one. Doing 4x 500m pieces as a dry run is also a good way to prove to yourself that you can handle a 2k test.

How to Pull a 2k Test and What It Feels Like

We are going to be honest here. There are few tests in life worse than a 2k test. A 2k will chew you up and spit you out if you aren't mentally prepared for it. Here is how we like to get through a 2k test.

If you're an experienced rower, you're going to have a target split in mind, but if you're a beginner, you have absolutely no idea. For beginners, we recommend being reasonable – holding a 2:30 split for ten minutes seems like something every reasonably fit person can do. If that seems too ambitious, try a 2:45 split. Aim for that the first time. If you do better, great; if you do worse, then there is room for improvement, but that seems like a good initial goal. Good luck! You're going to need it.

You want to lock in that target split in your brain. Some people write it on a sticky note and put it on the erg screen as a reminder. The first 250 – 350m of the erg test is pure adrenaline. If you go out too high, you will crash almost immediately thereafter, and you will be done before you even started. Instead, aim for the first ten better-than-split strokes to get going, and then lock in at your target split. Around 250 you will start to feel the pain in your legs as lactic acid builds up, and your lungs will begin to twinge with a bit of a burn. Your body is telling you that this is a terrible idea, that you're not ready, that you should be on a beach somewhere, but this is exactly the point where you have to convince yourself that you will finish at your goal. The next 750 meters are pure mental. Most people who quit 2k tests (and trust us, we've all been there) usually give up between the 600 – 1100 meter point. If your splits start going up and down and you can't hold consistently, you've got to refocus on your target number and convince your brain. Refuse to give up on that split, and get yourself into a good rhythm focusing on staying long and swinging into the finish.

As you head to the 1000m point, take a move – whether it be a 'Power 20' to drop your split for twenty strokes, or bumping your rating up two for ten to twenty strokes. This is as much psychological as it is physical, and it will take every ounce of will you've got to do it. Then with about 850 or so to go, you've got to get back into the groove of your target split. Your legs are in pain, your lungs are burning at this point, and every fiber of your being wants to give up, but tell yourself that you're more than halfway done, and there is no turning back now. You can try basic tactics like focusing on various technique points (sitting up tall, efficient breathing, staying long, pushing the heels down, etc.) for series of ten-stroke countdowns. Take it 100m by 100m or minute by minute. Whatever it takes to hold that target split. With about 250 to go, the end is in sight, and you'll want to drop the split down and take the rating up as you go, sprinting in the final meters.

Absolutely key throughout the entire thing is to stay consistent with your technique — don't get into any of the bad habits we talk about in this book, but especially not shortening up your stroke or throwing your back open too early. Good luck! (You're going to need it.)

Calculating Your Splits from a 2k

So you pulled a 2k test. You're going to divide your total time by four, and this will give you your 500 meter split. Let's say you pulled your 2k in 8:00. Your 2k pace would be a 2:00 split. Let's say you pulled your 2k in 9:20. Your 2k pace would be a 2:20 split. The good news is that you can completely avoid complicated math by plugging your numbers into one of the many online erg score calculators.

A Word on Weight Adjustment

As you might expect, heavier people can generally generate faster erg times than lighter ones. Many rowing coaches like to use what is known as 'weight adjustment' to account for the athlete's body weight when trying to build fast boats on the water. Heavy people have to pull their own weight, and sometimes a lighter person, even with a slower erg score, actually makes for a faster boat on the water. Even if you're exclusively an indoor rower, it is not a bad idea to plug your weight and erg times into a weight adjustment calculator to give you an idea of how you compare with others who might be heavier or lighter. There are a myriad of weight adjustment calculators available online.

GEAR FOR ROWING

What to Wear

You could probably erg in just about anything, but your ideal uniform for indoor rowing should be a pair of rowing trou (a fancy word for tight-fitting spandex shorts or tights) on the bottom and a t-shirt or tank on the top. Alternately, rowing in a unisuit (uni) designed for rowing is also highly comfortable, although it is hard to get off when you need to run to the bathroom between pieces. There are several companies that make clothing specifically for rowing, and we swear by JL Racing's rowing trou (short and long) and unis. JL's designs include compression where you want it and just a bit of padding on the rear. They come in an array of colors and styles for men and women, and the gender specific cuts are as flattering as you'll find anywhere. Boathouse Sports and Sew Sporty, along with other rowing-specific companies, also make specialized rowing gear.

We'll also put in a plug for compression tops as well, especially if you're carrying a little extra weight around your midsection. Anything that sucks you in has the advantage of helping you get the erg handle around the finish and away from the body easily and minimizes unwelcome clothing snags.

What Not to Wear

A short and incomplete list of things not to wear while erging:

- **Jewelry.** Avoid it all, but especially rings.

- **Gloves.** We get it; your hands get torn up, but real rowers don't wear gloves. Do it if you must, but don't let us see you wearing them.

- **Baggy basketball-style shorts.** Unless you want to get them caught in the tracks and potentially rip a hole in them and/or lose your pants, avoid these.

- **Baggy t-shirts.** Baggy t-shirts, especially those that bunch around the middle, are a bad idea because you can get your handle stuck trying to get the hands away from the body.

- **Bulky sweatshirts.** Bulky sweatshirts, especially with kangaroo-style pockets, can also cause the hands to get stuck by the body.

Other Rowing Gear

Here is another short list of things you might actually want while indoor rowing:

- **Water bottle.** This is an essential for any erg workout. We like the squeeze bottle type, so you can get a drink without taking your hands off the handle. Insulated squeeze bottles are even better.

- **Snacks.** If you're committed to long erg sessions, easy-to-eat food like protein bars and bananas are ideal for eating while erging and aren't too harsh on your stomach.

- **Small hand towel.** Great for wiping up sweat and snapping at other people erging around you.

- **Heart rate monitor.** Whether you're concerned about your heart, are training for elite performance or fall anywhere in between, a heart rate monitor can be a great tool.

- **Trash can.** Vomiting is an occasional side effect of indoor rowing. It is always good to be prepared for the worst-case scenario. Also, avoid eating burritos before erging, if you know what is good for you.

- **Mirror.** One of the best ways to improve your erging technique is to watch yourself in the mirror. Long mirrors designed for the back of bathroom doors can be ideal, although these are generally flimsy and can break if they are not affixed to a wall.

- **Video/Camera Setup.** Like a mirror, watching yourself on a video monitor or recording yourself to watch later is another great way to improve your technique. Clip on Go Pro style cameras are great for mounting on the erg screen for a front view.

- **Music.** Either through your mobile device or a boathouse speaker system, music is essential for erging.

- **Notebook.** A small notebook to capture scores and workouts is invaluable over the course of a winter training season and especially for new rowers just starting out.

- **White Board.** No boathouse, erg room or gym should go without a dry erase board or chalk board. This is perfect for displaying the day's workout, publically capturing the team's erg scores for the day (both good and embarrassing) and tallying points in team games and challenges. We buy our dry erase markers in bulk and still never to seem to have enough floating around the boathouse. Even if you're rowing by yourself in your garage, it's always nice to have a visual display of a complicated workout and maybe even an inspirational quote or two.

HOW TO USE THIS BOOK

Workout Basics

The following is a quick tutorial to decipher the workouts in this book.

Sample Workout

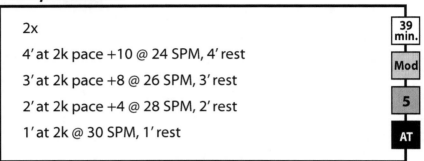

2x

4' at 2k pace +10 @ 24 SPM, 4' rest

3' at 2k pace +8 @ 26 SPM, 3' rest

2' at 2k pace +4 @ 28 SPM, 2' rest

1' at 2k @ 30 SPM, 1' rest

39 min.

Mod

5

AT

2x means two times. When you see that in front of a workout, it means you will run the entire thing twice. You might see workouts with 3x (three times), 4x (four times) and so on.

4' means four minutes, **3'** means three minutes and so on.

at 2k pace +10 means that you would take your average 2k split and add ten seconds to that. For example, if your average 2k split is 2:10, for this part of the workout you would pull four minutes at a 2:20 split. If your average 2k split was a 1:47, you would pull the four minutes at a 1:57 and so on. If you see something like at 2k pace -2, you would pull a split two seconds lower than your average 2k split. For example, if your average 2k pace was 1:54, your 2k pace -2 would be a 1:52 split. All of the workouts in this book are based on 2k or 6k average splits.

In order to pull at 2k pace +10, you would first need to calculate your 2k split by pulling a 2000m time trial as we describe in more detail at the beginning of this book.

@ 24 SPM means that you would pull this part of the workout at 24 strokes per minute. In this book you will find stroke ratings ranging from 16 SPM to 36 SPM.

4' rest means you would rest for four minutes after you pulled the first four-minute piece.

Here, for this sample workout, you would row for four minutes at 2k pace plus ten at 24 strokes per minute, rest for four minutes, pull three minutes at your 2k pace plus eight at 26 strokes per minute, rest for three minutes, pull two minutes at your 2k pace plus four at 28 strokes per minute, rest for two minutes, pull one minute at your 2k pace at 30 strokes per minute, rest for one minute, row for four minutes at 2k pace plus ten at 24 strokes per minute, rest for four minutes, pull three minutes at your 2k pace plus eight at 26 strokes per minute, rest for three minutes, pull two minutes at your 2k pace plus four at 28 strokes per minute, rest for two minutes and then pull one minute at your 2k pace at 30 strokes per minute.

Key to Workouts

The workouts in this book are coded with four pieces of information – time, level, pain rating and workout type. Understanding what these mean will improve your training and help you use this book.

Here is a basic explanation of each:

39 min.

Time. This is the **number of minutes** it will take you to complete the workout, including the warm up. Cool down time is not included.

Mod

Level. Each workout is coded as **Introductory, Moderate, Advanced or Team.** If you're just starting out, tackle at least a few of the Introductory workouts first. When these start to feel too easy, move on to the Moderate. Experienced rowers, especially rowing teams coming off the water for winter training should have no problem with the Advanced workouts, but should also include Introductory or Moderate workouts as needed. Team workouts are designed for groups of rowers.

5

Pain Rating. Pain rating is what we consider to be the amount of pain, on a scale of **1 to 10**, incurred for each workout. Introductory workouts have a pain rating of 1 to 3; moderate workouts have a pain rating from 4 to 5; and advanced workouts have a pain rating of 6 and above. Pain rating does not necessarily correlate to overall length of the workout, but longer workouts tend to have higher pain ratings. Pain rating is not an exact science, and we tended to gage pain rating based on how much our test rowers complained during the workouts. Also, keep in mind that pain does not necessarily equal gain. Doing a bunch of level 10 workouts all of the time can actually slow you down. Keep balance in mind.

Pain Rating Explained

1 Practically anybody off the street could get on an erg and do this.

2 You'll break a sweat and want to do something in addition to this workout.

3 You can tell people you worked out today, if you're into that sort of thing.

4 You'll feel like you accomplished something and might want to add something else to the workout.

5 You got a solid workout.

6 This workout was challenging. You'll definitely feel it tomorrow and at some point during the workout will want to quit.

7 At some point during this workout you'll want to quit, and you'll want to vomit. Or you may actually vomit.

8 At some point during this workout you'll contemplate your own mortality.

9 You will alternate among the stages of extreme leg burn, extreme lung burn, wanting to quit, wanting to vomit and thinking about all of the terrible things you'd like to do to the person who came up with it or forced you to do it.

10 Don't try this at home, kids. These are practically impossible unless you are a competitive athlete and mental beast. Category 10 workouts are generally stupid human tricks. You might be better off doing a handstand on a motorcycle.

Workout Type. All of the workouts in this book are coded **AN, O$_2$, AT or TR.** Here is a basic explanation of each:

AN is anaerobic exercise – speed work with very short, intense intervals. AN workouts are intervals of 30 – 90 seconds of work with much longer rest in between, typically at a 1:4 or 1:5 work to rest ratio. AN workouts are focused on building your speed and making you faster.

O$_2$ is aerobic exercise – steady state at moderate intensity. These workouts are designed to build your general fitness base. Typical O$_2$ workouts are things like steady state rowing for 30 minutes or more.

AT is anaerobic threshold – moderate workouts that have about 1:1 or 1:2 work to rest ratio. These are workouts where you should be able to row somewhere between a conversational pace and being totally out of breath. AT workouts are all about finding the threshold right before your body starts to really hurt (where you can't get rid of lactic acid). AT workouts are designed to build your capacity to row hard without hitting that lactic acid build up.

TR is transport – short, high intensity sprints. TR workouts generally have a 1:3 work to rest ratio. A typical TR workout is something like a 1000m sprint or a 2k erg test. The point of TR workouts is to force your body to deal with lactic acid build up and are as much mental as they are physical – you have to learn to row through the pain.

A note on workout types: Not every workout included in this book exactly fits the mold of the classic workout types listed above. Additionally, not every workout is exactly the same for every rower. For example, a workout that would be considered TR for a newer, less fit and less experienced rower might actually be an O$_2$ workout for a fit, elite level rower training for the Olympics. It is all relative to your fitness level, age and rowing experience. We tried to make the workouts in this book as universal as possible for rowers of all ages and abilities, and, as a result, some of it had to be generalized. Please consult with your coach or a sports trainer for a better assessment of your specific fitness goals and objectives.

Here is a basic pyramid for training programs:

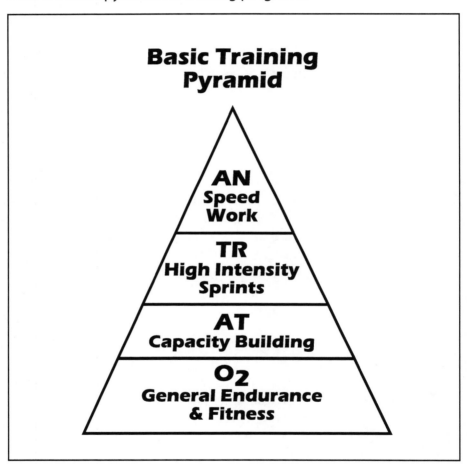

When designing a training program use the basic training pyramid as a guide. The largest part of the program should be O_2, general endurance and fitness. The next group of exercises should be AT, which are designed to build capacity. This will be followed by a smaller amount of (TR) high intensity sprints. AN speed workouts will comprise the smallest number of your workouts. We have provided two 14 week plans. You don't have to follow the training programs exactly, however, you will want to break up the intensity and avoid doing two TRs or two ANs back to back. Add an AT or an O_2 in between. You can also add an active rest day.

SAMPLE 14-WEEK TRAINING PROGRAMS

You can use the sample 14-week training programs below to peak for your target event (whether it is an indoor rowing race or on-the-water competition). We provide two general training programs based on the distance for your event. Each workout is marked O_2, AT, TR or AN, and you can fill in the details. For example, if Monday is an AT workout, you can select any AT workout in this book. If you're in the beginning stages, select an Introductory AT workout; if you're at an intermediate level, select a Moderate workout, and if you are an advanced rower, select an Advanced AT workout. You'll also want to keep in mind that advanced rowers should incorporate a healthy dose of introductory and moderate workouts into their training plans. Harder, longer workouts are not always better workouts. Go for a mix of levels for optimal training, even if you are an advanced rower.

To keep things fresh, try not to repeat workouts during your 14-week training program. On the Active Rest days, keep it light – swimming, walking, hiking, cycling – at a very light, low key pace. The other thing we'll mention is that if you're feeling tired or run down, it is fine (and in fact really a great idea) to take a day or two off. On the O_2 days you can also substitute erging with other steady state activities like running, biking or swimming.

Easy to use 14-week plans for a 2000M Sprint Race and for a 5000M-6000M Head Race follow on the next two pages.

BASIC 14-WEEK TRAINING PLAN FOR 2000M SPRINT RACE EVENT

Week	Sunday	Monday	Tuesday	Wednesday	Thursday	Friday	Saturday
1	Active Rest	O2	AT	O2	O2	O2	O2
2	Active Rest	AT	2k Test	O2	AT	O2	AT
3	Active Rest	AT	O2	AT	O2	AT	TR
4	Active Rest	O2	AT	O2	O2	AT	TR
5	Active Rest	O2	TR	O2	AT	O2	TR
6	Active Rest	O2	2k Test	O2	AT	TR	AT
7	Active Rest	AN	O2	AT	TR	O2	AT
8	Active Rest	AN	AT	TR	O2	O2	AT
9	Active Rest	AN	O2	O2	TR	O2	AT
10	Active Rest	AN	2K Test	O2	O2	AT	O2
11	Active Rest	AN	O2	TR	O2	AT	O2
12	Active Rest	AN	AT	TR	AT	O2	AT
13	Active Rest	AN	AT	TR	AT	TR	AN
14	Active Rest	TR	AT	AN	AN	O2	Race

BASIC 14-WEEK TRAINING PLAN FOR 5000M-6000M HEAD RACE EVENT

Week	Sunday	Monday	Tuesday	Wednesday	Thursday	Friday	Saturday
1	Active Rest	O2	O2	O2	O2	O2	O2
2	Active Rest	AT	6K Test	O2	AT	O2	AT
3	Active Rest	O2	O2	AT	O2	AT	O2
4	Active Rest	O2	O2	AT	O2	TR	O2
5	Active Rest	O2	AT	O2	TR	AT	O2
6	Active Rest	O2	6K Test	O2	TR	AT	O2
7	Active Rest	AT	TR	O2	TR	O2	AT
8	Active Rest	AT	TR	O2	TR	O2	AT
9	Active Rest	AT	TR	O2	AT	TR	O2
10	Active Rest	O2	6K Test	O2	TR	O2	AT
11	Active Rest	AN	O2	TR	O2	AT	O2
12	Active Rest	AN	O2	TR	O2	AT	O2
13	Active Rest	AN	AT	O2	AT	TR	AN
14	Active Rest	AN	AT	AN	AT	O2	Race

WORKOUTS

BASELINE WORKOUTS

If you're ready to get serious about erging, you need to test yourself periodically. Knowing your 2k and 6k test splits will help you use this book and maximize your training. We recommend doing a 2k test and a 6k test every 4-8 weeks and tracking your improvement.

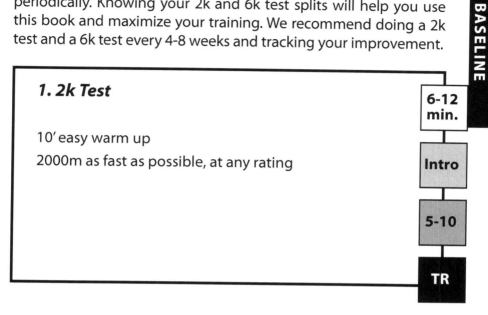

1. 2k Test

10' easy warm up

2000m as fast as possible, at any rating

6-12 min.

Intro

5-10

TR

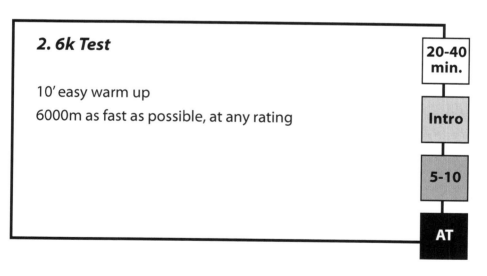

2. 6k Test

10' easy warm up

6000m as fast as possible, at any rating

20-40 min.

Intro

5-10

AT

45

SHORT ERG WORKOUTS

These workouts can be used for warm ups and when you don't have much time to work out.

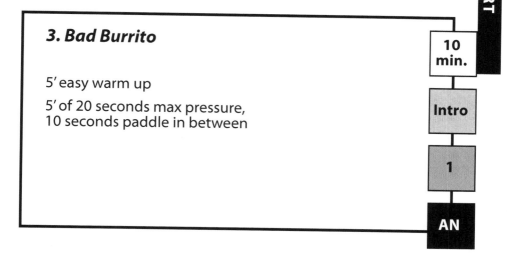

3. Bad Burrito

5' easy warm up

5' of 20 seconds max pressure,
10 seconds paddle in between

10 min.

Intro

1

AN

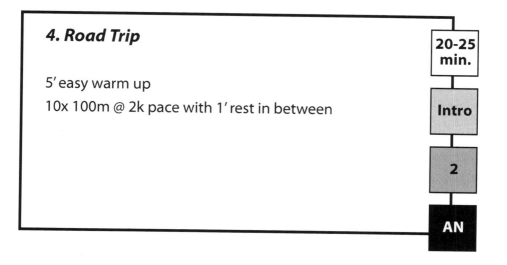

4. Road Trip

5' easy warm up

10x 100m @ 2k pace with 1' rest in between

20-25 min.

Intro

2

AN

47

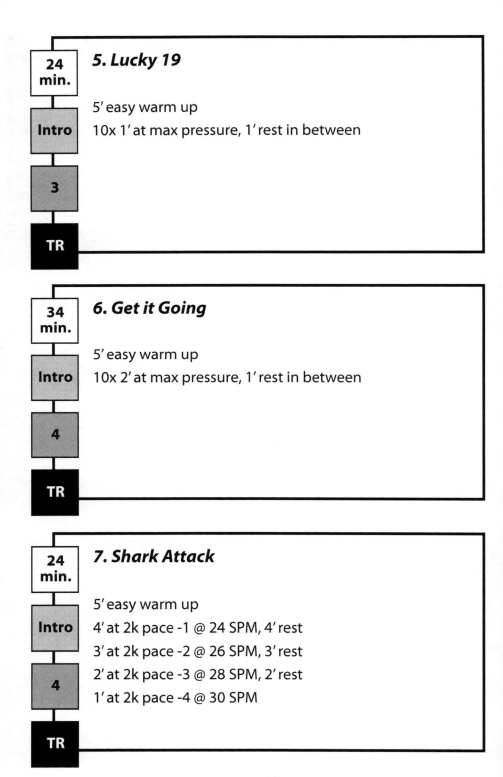

5. Lucky 19

24 min.

Intro

3

TR

5' easy warm up

10x 1' at max pressure, 1' rest in between

6. Get it Going

34 min.

Intro

4

TR

5' easy warm up

10x 2' at max pressure, 1' rest in between

7. Shark Attack

24 min.

Intro

4

TR

5' easy warm up

4' at 2k pace -1 @ 24 SPM, 4' rest

3' at 2k pace -2 @ 26 SPM, 3' rest

2' at 2k pace -3 @ 28 SPM, 2' rest

1' at 2k pace -4 @ 30 SPM

INTRODUCTORY WORKOUTS

These workouts are designed for new rowers, rowers recovery from injury, people with physical limitations and for days when you need an easier workout.

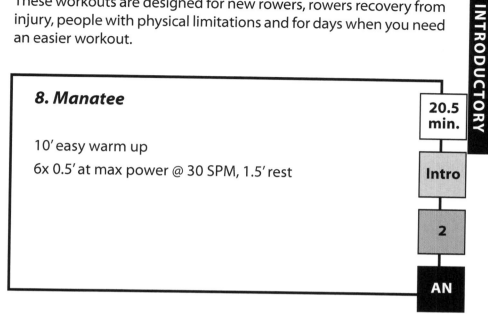

8. Manatee

10' easy warm up

6x 0.5' at max power @ 30 SPM, 1.5' rest

20.5 min.

Intro

2

AN

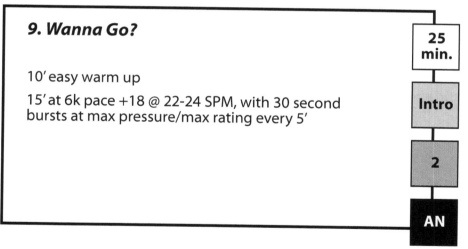

9. Wanna Go?

10' easy warm up

15' at 6k pace +18 @ 22-24 SPM, with 30 second bursts at max pressure/max rating every 5'

25 min.

Intro

2

AN

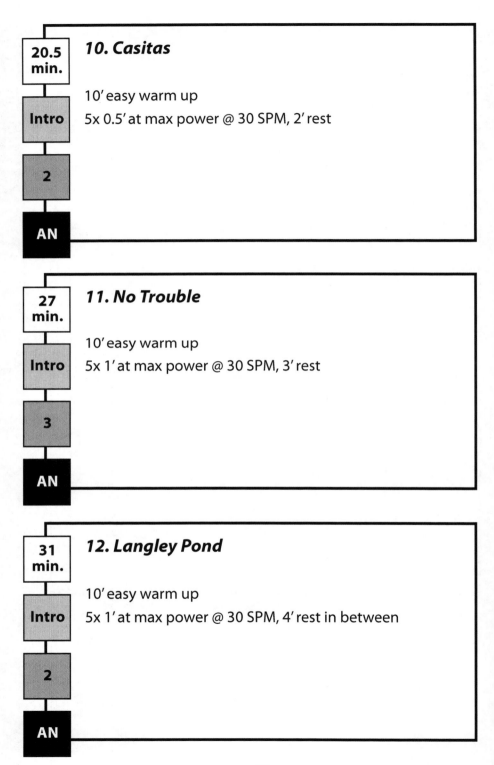

20.5 min.

Intro

2

AN

10. Casitas

10' easy warm up

5x 0.5' at max power @ 30 SPM, 2' rest

27 min.

Intro

3

AN

11. No Trouble

10' easy warm up

5x 1' at max power @ 30 SPM, 3' rest

31 min.

Intro

2

AN

12. Langley Pond

10' easy warm up

5x 1' at max power @ 30 SPM, 4' rest in between

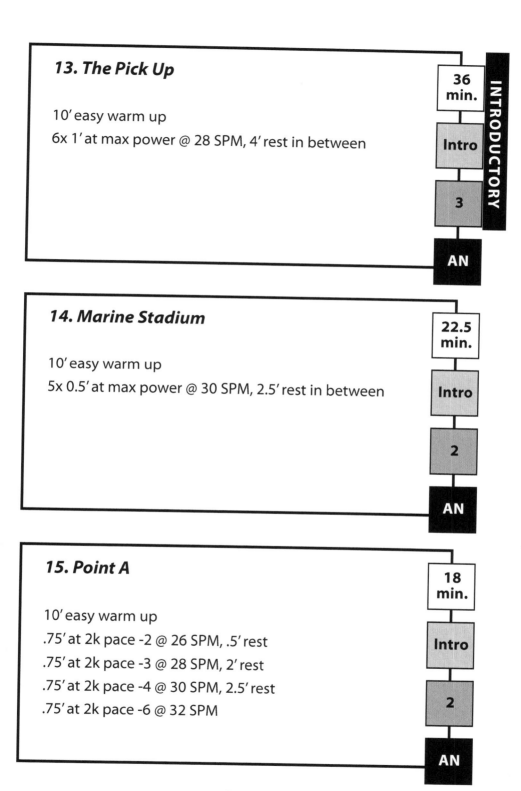

13. The Pick Up

10' easy warm up
6x 1' at max power @ 28 SPM, 4' rest in between

36 min.

Intro

3

AN

INTRODUCTORY

14. Marine Stadium

10' easy warm up
5x 0.5' at max power @ 30 SPM, 2.5' rest in between

22.5 min.

Intro

2

AN

15. Point A

10' easy warm up
.75' at 2k pace -2 @ 26 SPM, .5' rest
.75' at 2k pace -3 @ 28 SPM, 2' rest
.75' at 2k pace -4 @ 30 SPM, 2.5' rest
.75' at 2k pace -6 @ 32 SPM

18 min.

Intro

2

AN

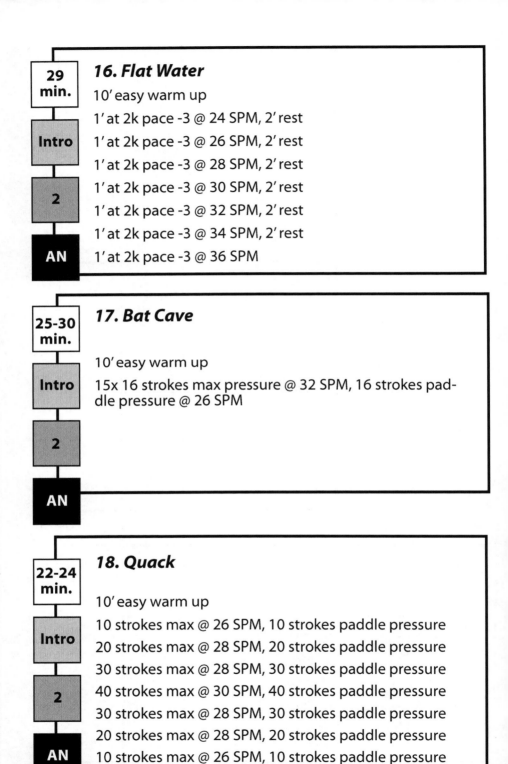

16. Flat Water

29 min.

Intro

2

AN

10' easy warm up

1' at 2k pace -3 @ 24 SPM, 2' rest

1' at 2k pace -3 @ 26 SPM, 2' rest

1' at 2k pace -3 @ 28 SPM, 2' rest

1' at 2k pace -3 @ 30 SPM, 2' rest

1' at 2k pace -3 @ 32 SPM, 2' rest

1' at 2k pace -3 @ 34 SPM, 2' rest

1' at 2k pace -3 @ 36 SPM

17. Bat Cave

25-30 min.

Intro

2

AN

10' easy warm up

15x 16 strokes max pressure @ 32 SPM, 16 strokes paddle pressure @ 26 SPM

18. Quack

22-24 min.

Intro

2

AN

10' easy warm up

10 strokes max @ 26 SPM, 10 strokes paddle pressure

20 strokes max @ 28 SPM, 20 strokes paddle pressure

30 strokes max @ 28 SPM, 30 strokes paddle pressure

40 strokes max @ 30 SPM, 40 strokes paddle pressure

30 strokes max @ 28 SPM, 30 strokes paddle pressure

20 strokes max @ 28 SPM, 20 strokes paddle pressure

10 strokes max @ 26 SPM, 10 strokes paddle pressure

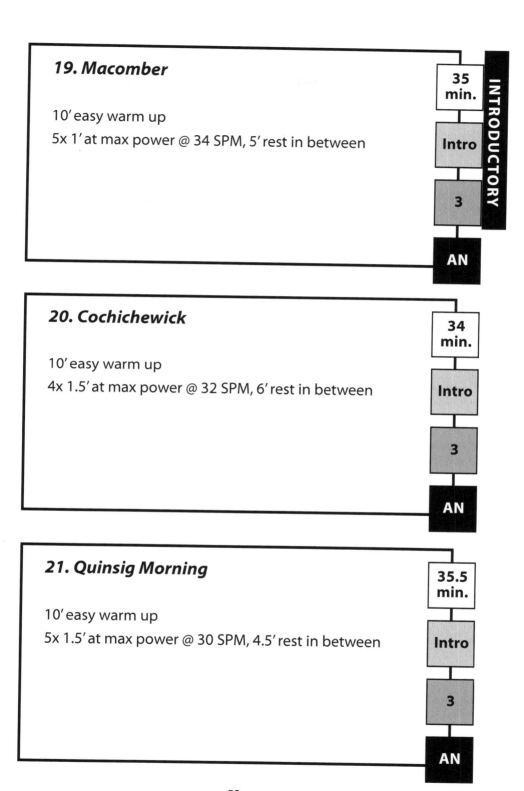

19. Macomber

10' easy warm up
5x 1' at max power @ 34 SPM, 5' rest in between

35 min.

Intro

3

AN

INTRODUCTORY

20. Cochichewick

10' easy warm up
4x 1.5' at max power @ 32 SPM, 6' rest in between

34 min.

Intro

3

AN

21. Quinsig Morning

10' easy warm up
5x 1.5' at max power @ 30 SPM, 4.5' rest in between

35.5 min.

Intro

3

AN

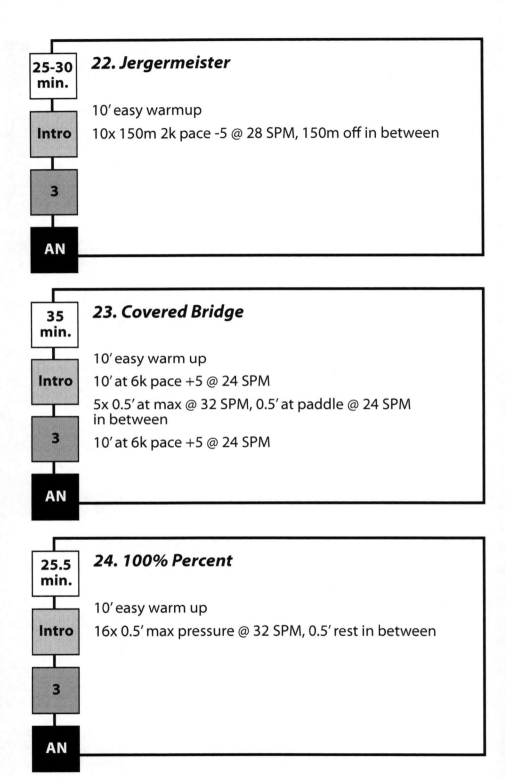

25-30 min.

Intro

3

AN

22. Jergermeister

10' easy warmup

10x 150m 2k pace -5 @ 28 SPM, 150m off in between

35 min.

Intro

3

AN

23. Covered Bridge

10' easy warm up

10' at 6k pace +5 @ 24 SPM

5x 0.5' at max @ 32 SPM, 0.5' at paddle @ 24 SPM in between

10' at 6k pace +5 @ 24 SPM

25.5 min.

Intro

3

AN

24. 100% Percent

10' easy warm up

16x 0.5' max pressure @ 32 SPM, 0.5' rest in between

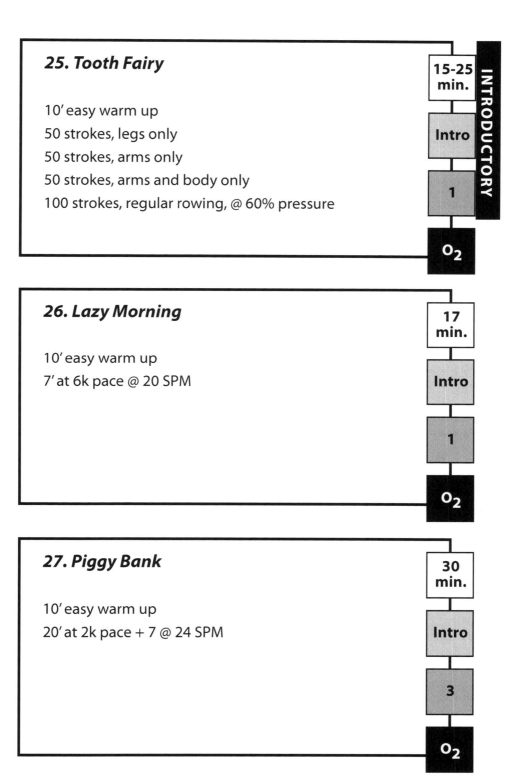

25. Tooth Fairy

10' easy warm up
50 strokes, legs only
50 strokes, arms only
50 strokes, arms and body only
100 strokes, regular rowing, @ 60% pressure

15-25 min.

Intro

1

O₂

INTRODUCTORY

26. Lazy Morning

10' easy warm up
7' at 6k pace @ 20 SPM

17 min.

Intro

1

O₂

27. Piggy Bank

10' easy warm up
20' at 2k pace + 7 @ 24 SPM

30 min.

Intro

3

O₂

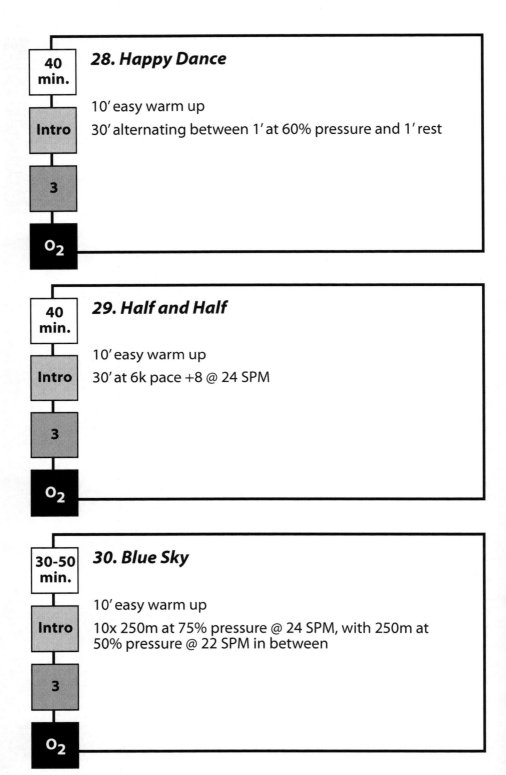

28. Happy Dance

40 min.

Intro

3

O₂

10' easy warm up

30' alternating between 1' at 60% pressure and 1' rest

29. Half and Half

40 min.

Intro

3

O₂

10' easy warm up

30' at 6k pace +8 @ 24 SPM

30. Blue Sky

30-50 min.

Intro

3

O₂

10' easy warm up

10x 250m at 75% pressure @ 24 SPM, with 250m at 50% pressure @ 22 SPM in between

31. Get a Grip

3' arms and body only rowing
3' half slide rowing
3' 3/4 slide rowing
3' full slide rowing at 50% pressure @ 18 SPM
3' full slide rowing at 75% pressure @ 20 SPM
3' full slide rowing at 6k pace @ 22 SPM

18 min.

Intro

1

O₂

INTRODUCTORY

32. Bright Idea

10' easy warm up
5' at 6k pace +10 @ 22 SPM, 2' rest
5' at 6k pace +8 @ 24 SPM, 2' rest
5' at 6k pace +6 @ 26 SPM, 2' rest

31 min.

Intro

2

O₂

33. Steady State Flow

10' easy warm up
30' at 6k pace +10 @ 22-24 SPM

40 min.

Intro

3

O₂

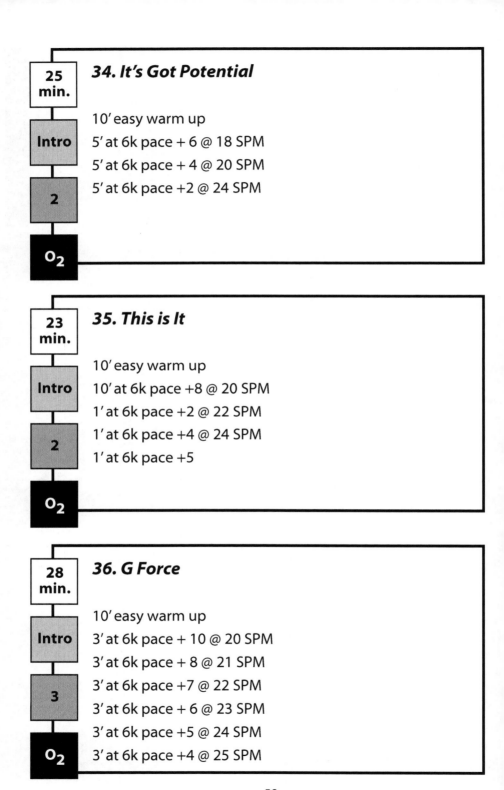

25 min.

Intro

2

O₂

34. It's Got Potential

10' easy warm up
5' at 6k pace + 6 @ 18 SPM
5' at 6k pace + 4 @ 20 SPM
5' at 6k pace +2 @ 24 SPM

23 min.

Intro

2

O₂

35. This is It

10' easy warm up
10' at 6k pace +8 @ 20 SPM
1' at 6k pace +2 @ 22 SPM
1' at 6k pace +4 @ 24 SPM
1' at 6k pace +5

28 min.

Intro

3

O₂

36. G Force

10' easy warm up
3' at 6k pace + 10 @ 20 SPM
3' at 6k pace + 8 @ 21 SPM
3' at 6k pace +7 @ 22 SPM
3' at 6k pace + 6 @ 23 SPM
3' at 6k pace +5 @ 24 SPM
3' at 6k pace +4 @ 25 SPM

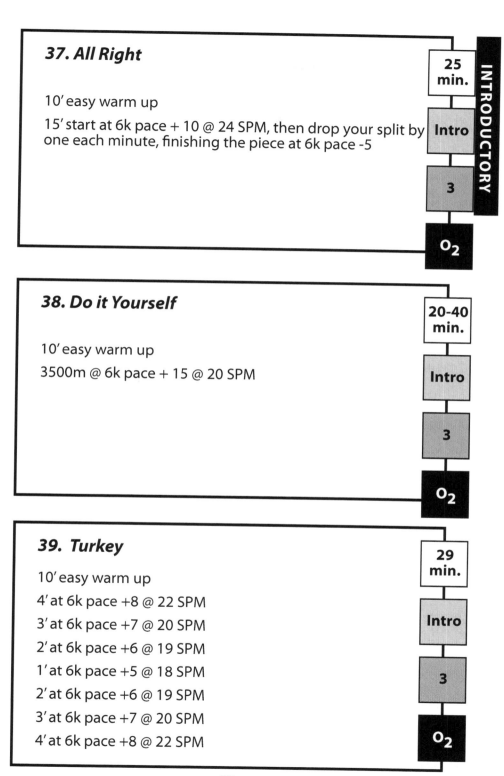

37. All Right

10' easy warm up

15' start at 6k pace + 10 @ 24 SPM, then drop your split by one each minute, finishing the piece at 6k pace -5

25 min.

Intro

3

O₂

INTRODUCTORY

38. Do it Yourself

10' easy warm up
3500m @ 6k pace + 15 @ 20 SPM

20-40 min.

Intro

3

O₂

39. Turkey

10' easy warm up
4' at 6k pace +8 @ 22 SPM
3' at 6k pace +7 @ 20 SPM
2' at 6k pace +6 @ 19 SPM
1' at 6k pace +5 @ 18 SPM
2' at 6k pace +6 @ 19 SPM
3' at 6k pace +7 @ 20 SPM
4' at 6k pace +8 @ 22 SPM

29 min.

Intro

3

O₂

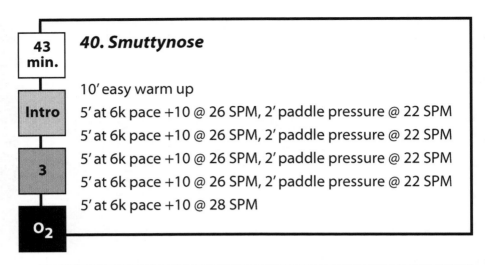

43 min.

Intro

3

O₂

40. Smuttynose

10' easy warm up
5' at 6k pace +10 @ 26 SPM, 2' paddle pressure @ 22 SPM
5' at 6k pace +10 @ 26 SPM, 2' paddle pressure @ 22 SPM
5' at 6k pace +10 @ 26 SPM, 2' paddle pressure @ 22 SPM
5' at 6k pace +10 @ 26 SPM, 2' paddle pressure @ 22 SPM
5' at 6k pace +10 @ 28 SPM

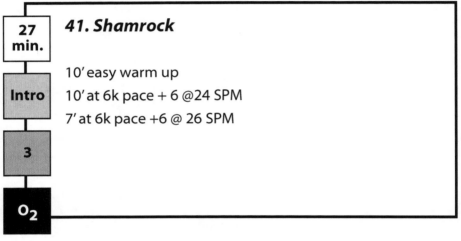

27 min.

Intro

3

O₂

41. Shamrock

10' easy warm up
10' at 6k pace + 6 @24 SPM
7' at 6k pace +6 @ 26 SPM

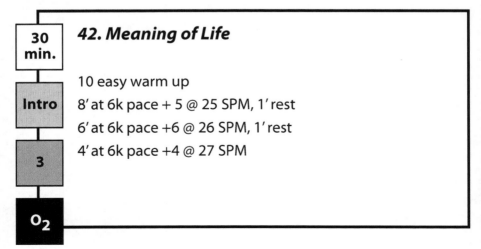

30 min.

Intro

3

O₂

42. Meaning of Life

10 easy warm up
8' at 6k pace + 5 @ 25 SPM, 1' rest
6' at 6k pace +6 @ 26 SPM, 1' rest
4' at 6k pace +4 @ 27 SPM

43. Anacostia

10' easy warm up
26' at 6k pace +4 @ 18 SPM

36 min.

Intro

3

O₂

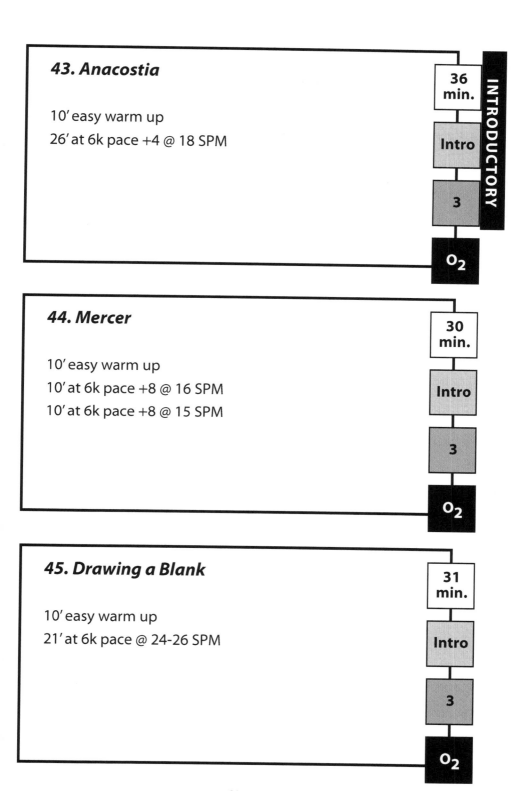

INTRODUCTORY

44. Mercer

10' easy warm up
10' at 6k pace +8 @ 16 SPM
10' at 6k pace +8 @ 15 SPM

30 min.

Intro

3

O₂

45. Drawing a Blank

10' easy warm up
21' at 6k pace @ 24-26 SPM

31 min.

Intro

3

O₂

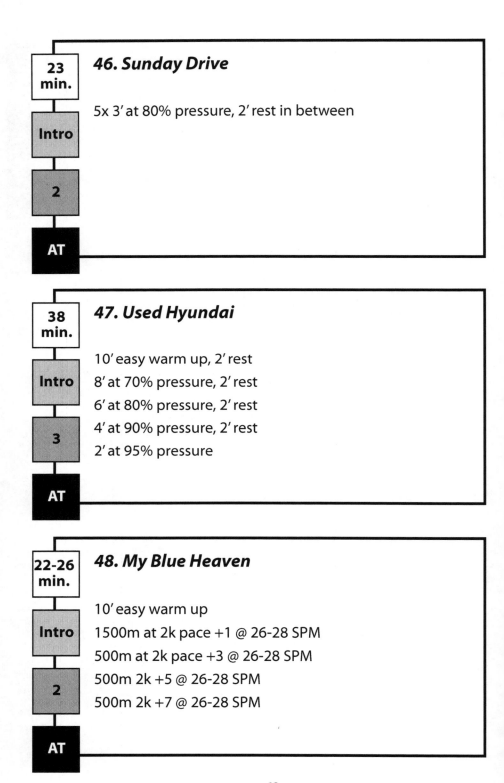

23 min.

Intro

2

AT

46. Sunday Drive

5x 3' at 80% pressure, 2' rest in between

38 min.

Intro

3

AT

47. Used Hyundai

10' easy warm up, 2' rest
8' at 70% pressure, 2' rest
6' at 80% pressure, 2' rest
4' at 90% pressure, 2' rest
2' at 95% pressure

22-26 min.

Intro

2

AT

48. My Blue Heaven

10' easy warm up
1500m at 2k pace +1 @ 26-28 SPM
500m at 2k pace +3 @ 26-28 SPM
500m 2k +5 @ 26-28 SPM
500m 2k +7 @ 26-28 SPM

49. Summer Daze

10' easy warm up
750m at 2k pace @ 28 SPM, 3' rest
750m at 2k pace @ 26 SPM, 3' rest
750m at 2k pace @ 28 SPM

25-28 min.

Intro

2

AT

INTRODUCTORY

50. Who Knew?

10' easy warm up
500m at 2k pace @ 28 SPM, 2' rest
500m at 2k pace -3 @ 28 SPM, 2' rest
500m at 2k pace -6 @ 28 SPM

16-20 min.

Intro

2

AT

51. East Dam

10' easy warm up
1500m at 2k pace + 5 @ 26 SPM, 3' rest
3x 500m at 2k pace +5 @ 28 SPM, 1' rest in between

28-32 min.

Intro

2

AT

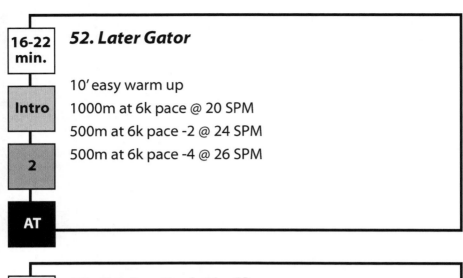

16-22 min.

Intro

2

AT

52. Later Gator

10' easy warm up

1000m at 6k pace @ 20 SPM

500m at 6k pace -2 @ 24 SPM

500m at 6k pace -4 @ 26 SPM

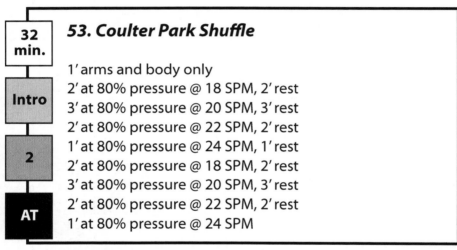

32 min.

Intro

2

AT

53. Coulter Park Shuffle

1' arms and body only

2' at 80% pressure @ 18 SPM, 2' rest

3' at 80% pressure @ 20 SPM, 3' rest

2' at 80% pressure @ 22 SPM, 2' rest

1' at 80% pressure @ 24 SPM, 1' rest

2' at 80% pressure @ 18 SPM, 2' rest

3' at 80% pressure @ 20 SPM, 3' rest

2' at 80% pressure @ 22 SPM, 2' rest

1' at 80% pressure @ 24 SPM

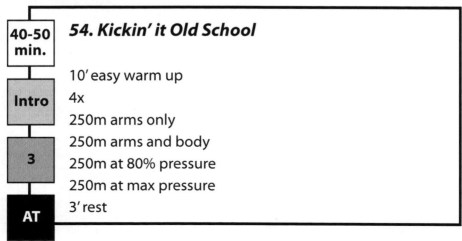

40-50 min.

Intro

3

AT

54. Kickin' it Old School

10' easy warm up

4x

250m arms only

250m arms and body

250m at 80% pressure

250m at max pressure

3' rest

55. Over Easy

500m half slide rowing at paddle pressure
1000m full slide at 50% pressure @ 18 SPM
1000m full slide at 75% pressure @ 20 SPM
500m full slide at 6k pace @ 22 SPM

20-25 min.

Intro

3

AT

INTRODUCTORY

56. Simple Pyramid

10' easy warm up
1' at 6k pace +10 @ 16 SPM, 1' rest
2' at 6k pace +8 @ 18 SPM, 2' rest
3' at 6k pace + 6 @ 20 SPM, 3' rest
4' at 6k pace +4 @ 22 SPM, 4' rest
3' at 6k pace +6 @ 20 SPM, 3' rest
2' at 6k pace +8 @ 18 SPM, 2' rest
1' at 6k pace +10 @ 16 SPM

41 min.

Intro

3

AT

57. Easy Does It

10' easy warm up
10x 1' at 6k pace @ 22 SPM, 1' off in between

29 min.

Intro

2

AT

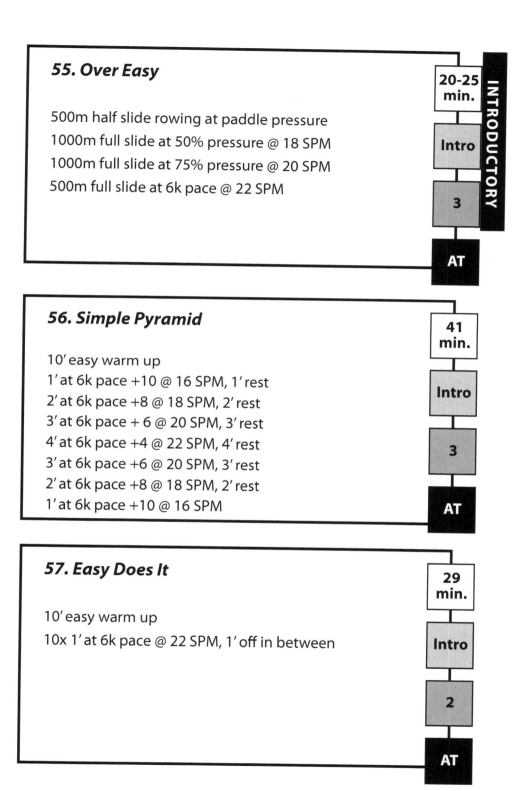

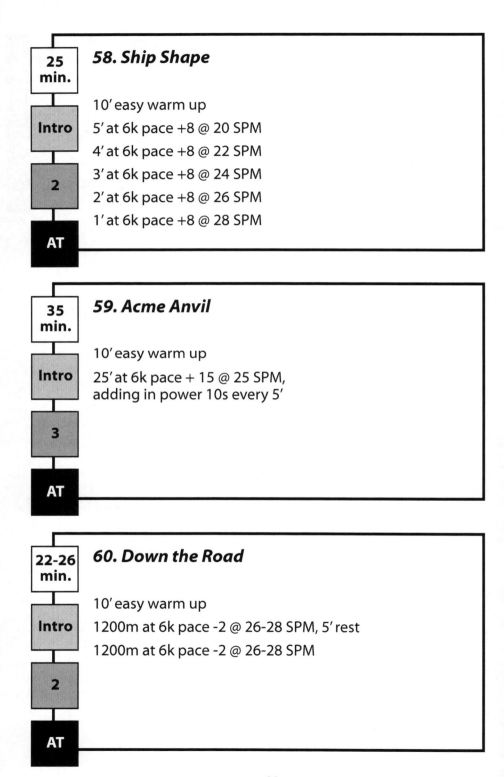

25 min.

Intro

2

AT

58. Ship Shape

10' easy warm up
5' at 6k pace +8 @ 20 SPM
4' at 6k pace +8 @ 22 SPM
3' at 6k pace +8 @ 24 SPM
2' at 6k pace +8 @ 26 SPM
1' at 6k pace +8 @ 28 SPM

35 min.

Intro

3

AT

59. Acme Anvil

10' easy warm up
25' at 6k pace + 15 @ 25 SPM,
adding in power 10s every 5'

22-26 min.

Intro

2

AT

60. Down the Road

10' easy warm up
1200m at 6k pace -2 @ 26-28 SPM, 5' rest
1200m at 6k pace -2 @ 26-28 SPM

61. Port Royal

10' easy warm up
2x 8' at 2k pace +14 @ 24 SPM, 8' rest in between

34 min.

Intro

3

AT

INTRODUCTORY

62. It'll Cost Ya

10' easy warm up
1000m at 6k pace @ 25 SPM, 2' rest
500m at 6k pace -2 @ 27 SPM, 2' rest
250m at 2k pace @ 32 SPM

21 min.

Intro

3

AT

63. Ebb Tide

10' easy warm up
4x 2.5' at 6k pace @ 24-26 SPM, 2.5' rest

27.5 min.

Intro

2

AT

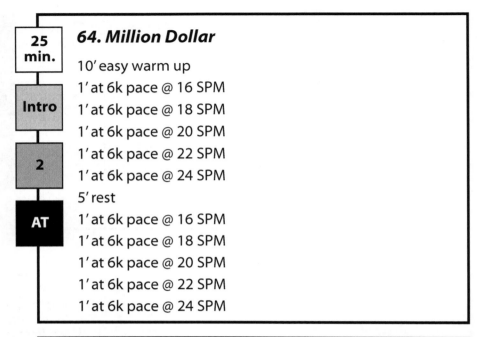

64. Million Dollar

25 min.

Intro

2

AT

10' easy warm up
1' at 6k pace @ 16 SPM
1' at 6k pace @ 18 SPM
1' at 6k pace @ 20 SPM
1' at 6k pace @ 22 SPM
1' at 6k pace @ 24 SPM
5' rest
1' at 6k pace @ 16 SPM
1' at 6k pace @ 18 SPM
1' at 6k pace @ 20 SPM
1' at 6k pace @ 22 SPM
1' at 6k pace @ 24 SPM

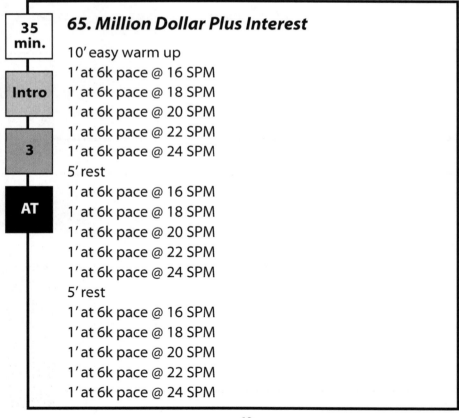

65. Million Dollar Plus Interest

35 min.

Intro

3

AT

10' easy warm up
1' at 6k pace @ 16 SPM
1' at 6k pace @ 18 SPM
1' at 6k pace @ 20 SPM
1' at 6k pace @ 22 SPM
1' at 6k pace @ 24 SPM
5' rest
1' at 6k pace @ 16 SPM
1' at 6k pace @ 18 SPM
1' at 6k pace @ 20 SPM
1' at 6k pace @ 22 SPM
1' at 6k pace @ 24 SPM
5' rest
1' at 6k pace @ 16 SPM
1' at 6k pace @ 18 SPM
1' at 6k pace @ 20 SPM
1' at 6k pace @ 22 SPM
1' at 6k pace @ 24 SPM

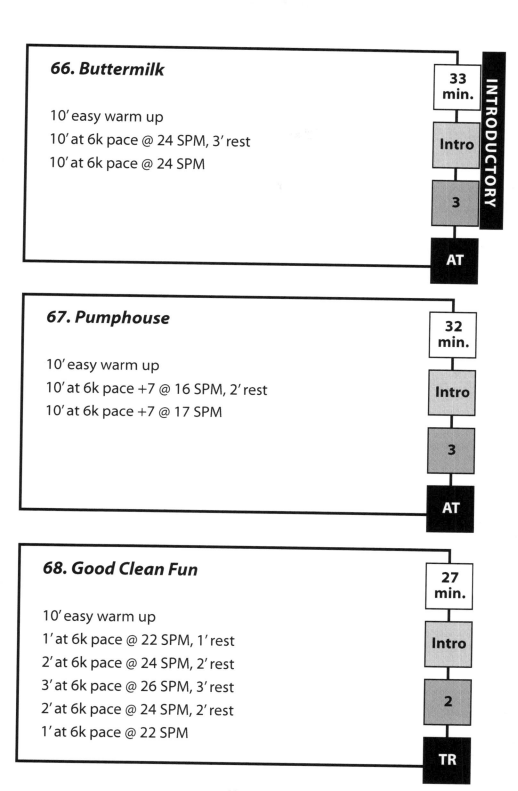

66. Buttermilk

10' easy warm up
10' at 6k pace @ 24 SPM, 3' rest
10' at 6k pace @ 24 SPM

33 min.

Intro

3

AT

INTRODUCTORY

67. Pumphouse

10' easy warm up
10' at 6k pace +7 @ 16 SPM, 2' rest
10' at 6k pace +7 @ 17 SPM

32 min.

Intro

3

AT

68. Good Clean Fun

10' easy warm up
1' at 6k pace @ 22 SPM, 1' rest
2' at 6k pace @ 24 SPM, 2' rest
3' at 6k pace @ 26 SPM, 3' rest
2' at 6k pace @ 24 SPM, 2' rest
1' at 6k pace @ 22 SPM

27 min.

Intro

2

TR

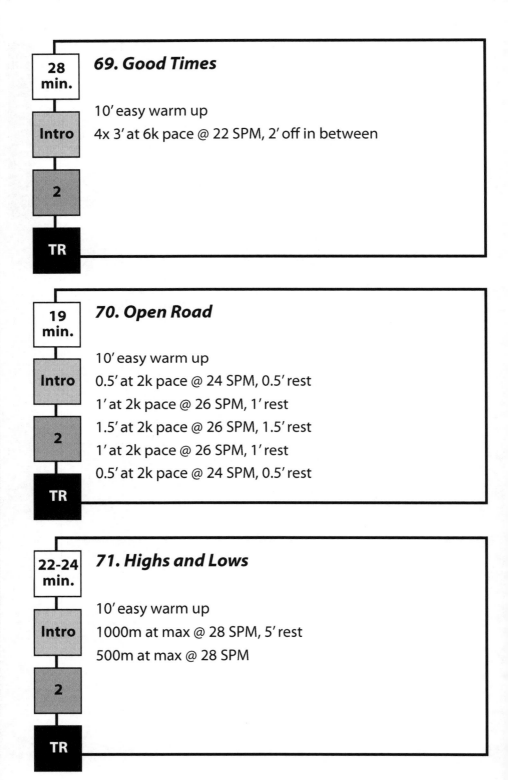

28 min.

Intro

2

TR

69. Good Times

10' easy warm up
4x 3' at 6k pace @ 22 SPM, 2' off in between

19 min.

Intro

2

TR

70. Open Road

10' easy warm up
0.5' at 2k pace @ 24 SPM, 0.5' rest
1' at 2k pace @ 26 SPM, 1' rest
1.5' at 2k pace @ 26 SPM, 1.5' rest
1' at 2k pace @ 26 SPM, 1' rest
0.5' at 2k pace @ 24 SPM, 0.5' rest

22-24 min.

Intro

2

TR

71. Highs and Lows

10' easy warm up
1000m at max @ 28 SPM, 5' rest
500m at max @ 28 SPM

72. Chatham

10' easy warm up
5x 300m at 2k pace -3 @ 30 SPM, 300 paddle @ 20 SPM

28-32 min.

Intro

3

TR

INTRODUCTORY

73. Having Fun

10' easy warm up
10x 1' at 6k pace -4 @ 24 SPM, 1' rest

29 min.

Intro

2

TR

74. Lucky Charm

10' easy warm up
5x 0.5' at 6k pace -6 @20 SPM, 1.5' rest in between
5x 1' at 6k pace -4 @23 SPM, 2' rest in between

33 min.

Intro

3

TR

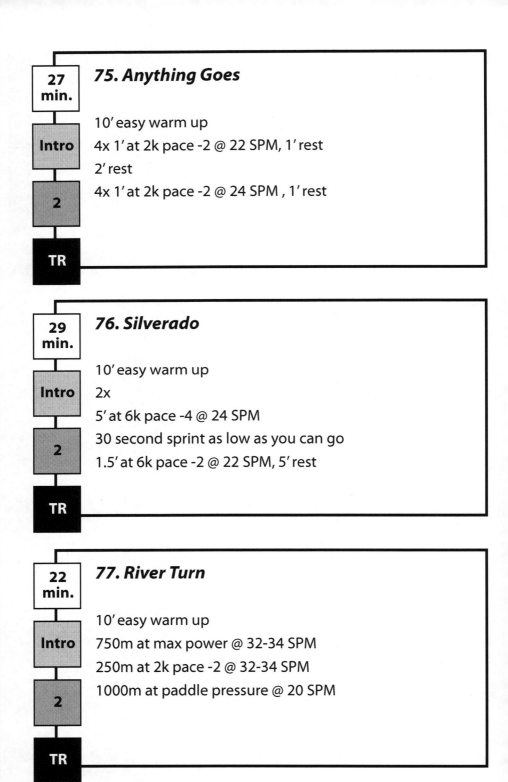

27 min.

Intro

2

TR

75. Anything Goes

10' easy warm up
4x 1' at 2k pace -2 @ 22 SPM, 1' rest
2' rest
4x 1' at 2k pace -2 @ 24 SPM , 1' rest

29 min.

Intro

2

TR

76. Silverado

10' easy warm up
2x
5' at 6k pace -4 @ 24 SPM
30 second sprint as low as you can go
1.5' at 6k pace -2 @ 22 SPM, 5' rest

22 min.

Intro

2

TR

77. River Turn

10' easy warm up
750m at max power @ 32-34 SPM
250m at 2k pace -2 @ 32-34 SPM
1000m at paddle pressure @ 20 SPM

78. Thursday Night

10' easy warm up
2' at 6k pace @ 28 SPM
1' at 2k pace -3 @ 30 SPM
2' at 6k pace @ 28 SPM
1' at 2k pace @ 30 SPM
2' at 6k pace @ 28 SPM
1' at 2k pace -3 @ 30 SPM

19 min.

Intro

2

TR

INTRODUCTORY

79. Bogeyman

10' easy warm up

3x 500m at 2k pace -2 @ 28 SPM, 30 strokes off in between

18-22 min.

Intro

2

TR

80. Bend in the Road

10' easy warm up

5 x 3' at 2k pace +4 @ 24-26 SPM, 1' rest in between

29 min.

Intro

3

TR

73

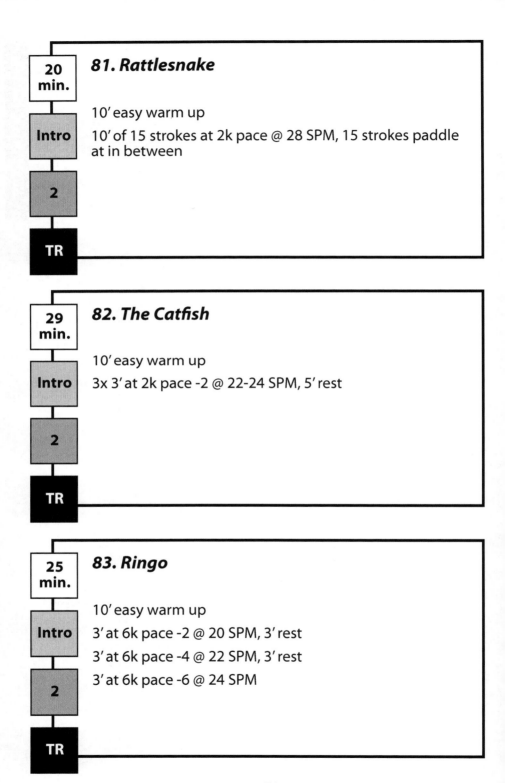

20 min.

Intro

2

TR

81. Rattlesnake

10' easy warm up

10' of 15 strokes at 2k pace @ 28 SPM, 15 strokes paddle at in between

29 min.

Intro

2

TR

82. The Catfish

10' easy warm up

3x 3' at 2k pace -2 @ 22-24 SPM, 5' rest

25 min.

Intro

2

TR

83. Ringo

10' easy warm up

3' at 6k pace -2 @ 20 SPM, 3' rest

3' at 6k pace -4 @ 22 SPM, 3' rest

3' at 6k pace -6 @ 24 SPM

84. Calhoun Beach

10' easy warm up
500m at max pressure @ 28 SPM, 1' rest
400m at max pressure @ 29 SPM, 1' rest
300m at max pressure @30 SPM, 1' rest
200m at max pressure @ 31 SPM, 1' rest
100m at max pressure @ 32 SPM

20-22 min.

Intro

3

TR

INTRODUCTORY

85. At Altitude

10' easy warm up
500m at max pressure @ 28 SPM, 1' rest
500m at max pressure @ 29 SPM, 1' rest
500m at max pressure @ 30 SPM, 1' rest

19 min.

Intro

3

TR

86. Glenmore

10' easy warm up
7x 45 strokes max pressure, max rating, 15 strokes off

28-32 min.

Intro

3

TR

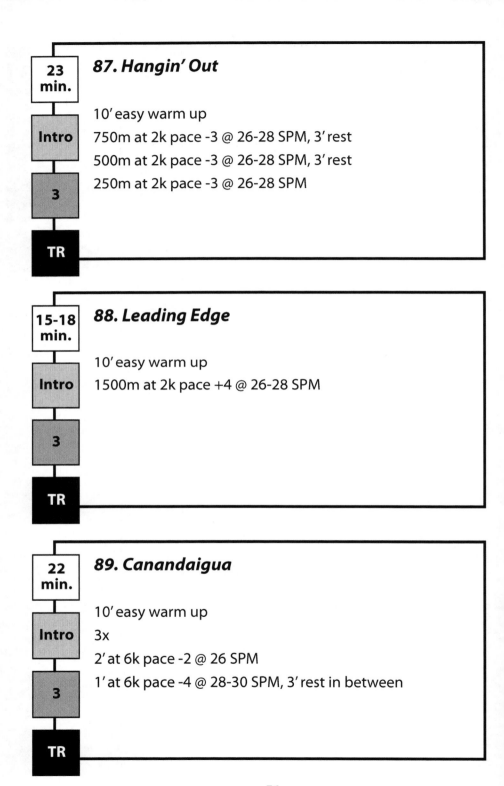

87. Hangin' Out

23 min.

Intro

3

TR

10' easy warm up
750m at 2k pace -3 @ 26-28 SPM, 3' rest
500m at 2k pace -3 @ 26-28 SPM, 3' rest
250m at 2k pace -3 @ 26-28 SPM

88. Leading Edge

15-18 min.

Intro

3

TR

10' easy warm up
1500m at 2k pace +4 @ 26-28 SPM

89. Canandaigua

22 min.

Intro

3

TR

10' easy warm up
3x
2' at 6k pace -2 @ 26 SPM
1' at 6k pace -4 @ 28-30 SPM, 3' rest in between

90. Om

10' easy warm up
1' at 6k pace -8 @ 26 SPM, 1' rest
2' at 6k pace -6 @ 26 SPM, 1' rest
3' at 6k pace -4 @ 26 SPM, 1' rest
5' at 6k pace -2 @

24 min.

Intro

3

TR

INTRODUCTORY

MODERATE INTENSITY WORKOUTS

These workouts are for more experienced rowers and provide an effective, moderate workout. Almost all of the workouts in this section can be completed in an hour or less. We recommend doing all moderate intensity erg workouts with what we call '10' easy warm up' at the beginning. This includes rowing at 25% pressure for the first few minutes and steadily building to a light, comfortable, steady state rowing, no more than 75% of your max pressure. After the workout, spend at least 5 minutes on the erg in a light cool down.

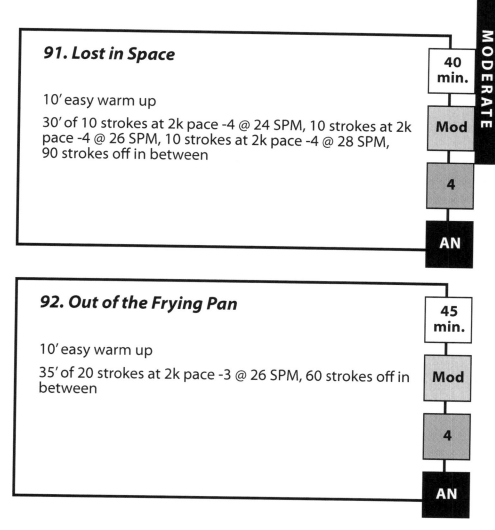

91. Lost in Space

10' easy warm up

30' of 10 strokes at 2k pace -4 @ 24 SPM, 10 strokes at 2k pace -4 @ 26 SPM, 10 strokes at 2k pace -4 @ 28 SPM, 90 strokes off in between

40 min.

Mod

4

AN

MODERATE

92. Out of the Frying Pan

10' easy warm up

35' of 20 strokes at 2k pace -3 @ 26 SPM, 60 strokes off in between

45 min.

Mod

4

AN

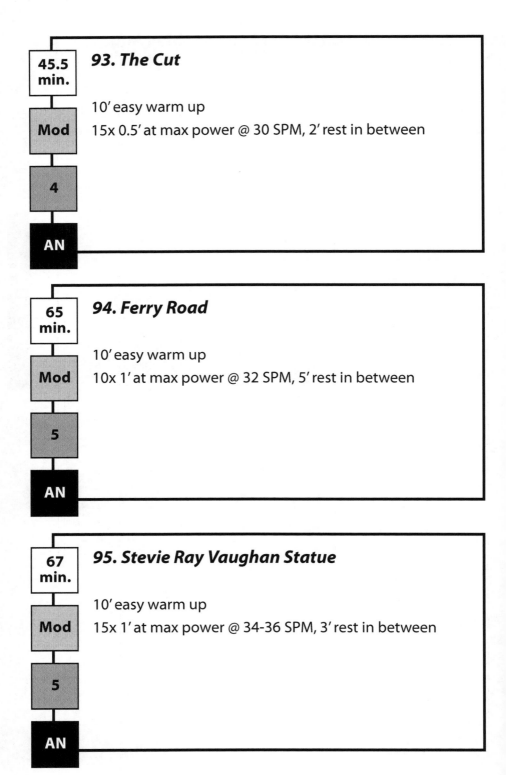

45.5 min.

Mod

4

AN

93. The Cut

10' easy warm up

15x 0.5' at max power @ 30 SPM, 2' rest in between

65 min.

Mod

5

AN

94. Ferry Road

10' easy warm up

10x 1' at max power @ 32 SPM, 5' rest in between

67 min.

Mod

5

AN

95. Stevie Ray Vaughan Statue

10' easy warm up

15x 1' at max power @ 34-36 SPM, 3' rest in between

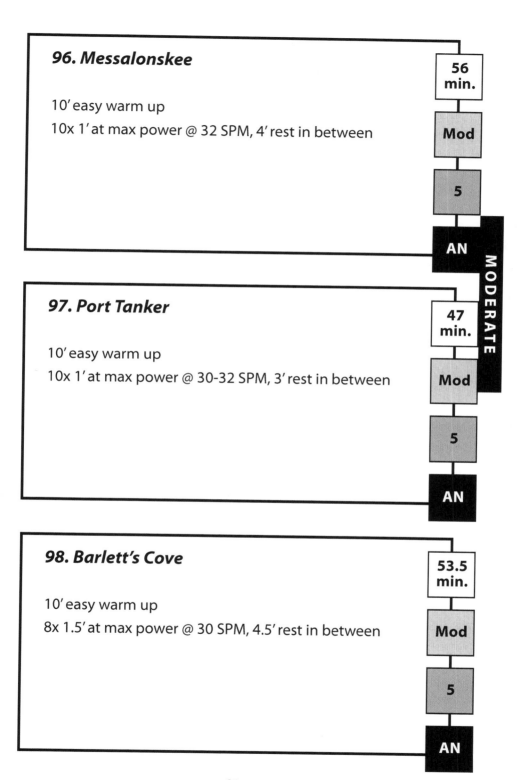

96. Messalonskee

10' easy warm up
10x 1' at max power @ 32 SPM, 4' rest in between

56 min.

Mod

5

AN

97. Port Tanker

10' easy warm up
10x 1' at max power @ 30-32 SPM, 3' rest in between

47 min.

Mod

5

AN

MODERATE

98. Barlett's Cove

10' easy warm up
8x 1.5' at max power @ 30 SPM, 4.5' rest in between

53.5 min.

Mod

5

AN

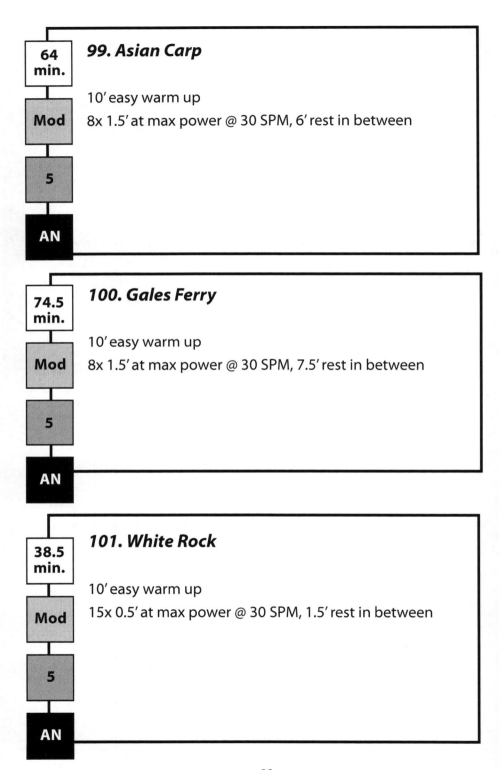

64 min.

Mod

5

AN

99. Asian Carp

10' easy warm up

8x 1.5' at max power @ 30 SPM, 6' rest in between

74.5 min.

Mod

5

AN

100. Gales Ferry

10' easy warm up

8x 1.5' at max power @ 30 SPM, 7.5' rest in between

38.5 min.

Mod

5

AN

101. White Rock

10' easy warm up

15x 0.5' at max power @ 30 SPM, 1.5' rest in between

102. Merced Madness

10' easy warm up

15x 0.5' at max power @ 30 SPM, 2.5' rest in between

52.5 min.

Mod

5

AN

103. Launch Lizard

10' easy warm up

15 x 16 strokes max pressure @ 32 SPM, 16 strokes paddle pressure @ 26 SPM

3' rest

15 x 16 strokes max pressure @ 32 SPM, 16 strokes paddle pressure @ 26 SPM

40-50 min.

Mod

4

AN

MODERATE

104. Broken Rigger

10' easy warm up

3x

10 strokes max @ 26 SPM, 10 strokes paddle pressure

20 strokes max @ 28 SPM, 20 strokes paddle pressure

30 strokes max @28 SPM, 30 strokes paddle pressure

40 strokes max @ 30 SPM, 40 strokes paddle pressure

30 strokes max @ 28 SPM, 30 strokes paddle pressure

20 strokes max @ 28 SPM, 20 strokes paddle pressure

10 strokes max @ 26 SPM, 10 strokes paddle pressure

46-50 min.

Mod

5

AN

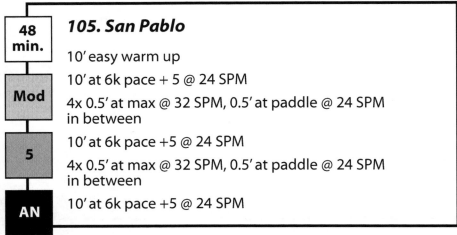

48 min.

Mod

5

AN

105. San Pablo

10' easy warm up

10' at 6k pace + 5 @ 24 SPM

4x 0.5' at max @ 32 SPM, 0.5' at paddle @ 24 SPM in between

10' at 6k pace +5 @ 24 SPM

4x 0.5' at max @ 32 SPM, 0.5' at paddle @ 24 SPM in between

10' at 6k pace +5 @ 24 SPM

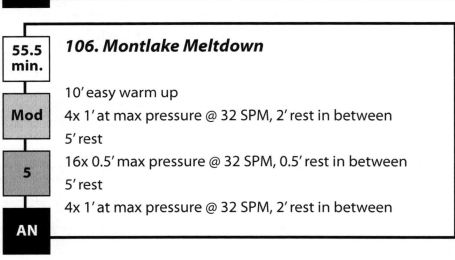

55.5 min.

Mod

5

AN

106. Montlake Meltdown

10' easy warm up

4x 1' at max pressure @ 32 SPM, 2' rest in between

5' rest

16x 0.5' max pressure @ 32 SPM, 0.5' rest in between

5' rest

4x 1' at max pressure @ 32 SPM, 2' rest in between

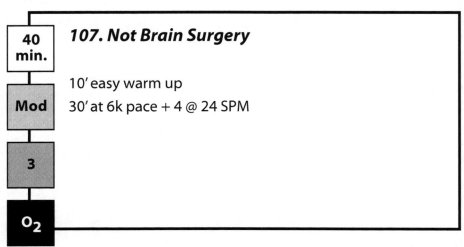

40 min.

Mod

3

O₂

107. Not Brain Surgery

10' easy warm up

30' at 6k pace + 4 @ 24 SPM

108. Get Loose

10' easy warm up
6' at 6k pace +10 @ 24 SPM, 1' rest
6' at 6k pace +8 @ 24 SPM, 1' rest
6' at 6k pace +6 @ 26 SPM, 1' rest
6' at 6k pace +6 @ 24 SPM

37 min.

Mod

3

O₂

109. 72nd Street Bridge

10' easy warm up
5' at 6k pace +10 @ 22 SPM, 3' rest
5' at 6k pace +8 @ 26 SPM, 3' rest
5' at 6k pace +10 @ 22 SPM, 3' rest
5' at 6k pace +8 @ 26 SPM, 3' rest
5' at 6k pace +10 @ 22 SPM, 3' rest
5' at 6k pace +10 @ 22 SPM, 3' rest
5' at 6k pace +8 @ 26 SPM

47 min.

Mod

3

O₂

MODERATE

110. Have At It

10' easy warm up
5' at 6k pace +12 @ 20 SPM, 2' rest
5' at 6k pace +10 @ 22 SPM, 2' rest
5' at 6k pace +8 @ 24 SPM, 2' rest
5' at 6k pace +6 @ 26 SPM, 2' rest
5' at 6k pace +4 @ 28 SPM

43 min.

Mod

4

O₂

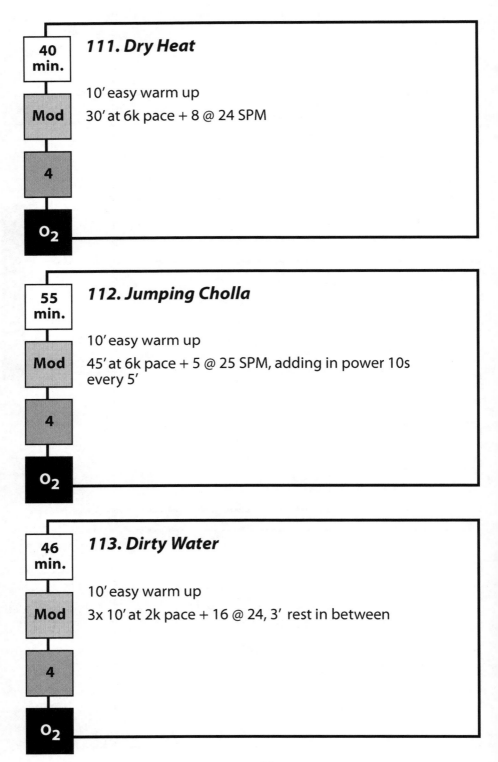

40 min.

Mod

4

O₂

111. Dry Heat

10' easy warm up
30' at 6k pace + 8 @ 24 SPM

55 min.

Mod

4

O₂

112. Jumping Cholla

10' easy warm up
45' at 6k pace + 5 @ 25 SPM, adding in power 10s every 5'

46 min.

Mod

4

O₂

113. Dirty Water

10' easy warm up
3x 10' at 2k pace + 16 @ 24, 3' rest in between

114. Slam Dunk

10' easy warm up
1000m at 6k pace +13 @ 20 SPM
1500m at 6k pace +12 @ 22 SPM
1500m at 6k pace +10 @ 24 SPM
500m at 6k pace +8 @ 26 SPM
500m at 6k pace +6 @ 28 SPM

30-38 min.

Mod

4

O₂

115. Green Mountain

10' easy warm up
25' at 6k pace + 6 @ 25 SPM

35 min.

Mod

4

O₂

MODERATE

116. Half Marathon

21,000 meters total, starting with warmup,
building intensity and rating as you go

75-90 min.

Mod

5

O₂

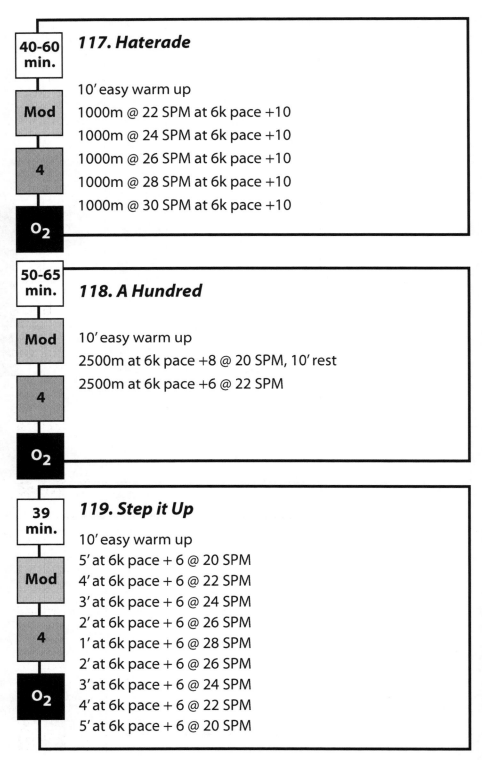

40-60 min.

Mod

4

O₂

117. Haterade

10' easy warm up
1000m @ 22 SPM at 6k pace +10
1000m @ 24 SPM at 6k pace +10
1000m @ 26 SPM at 6k pace +10
1000m @ 28 SPM at 6k pace +10
1000m @ 30 SPM at 6k pace +10

50-65 min.

Mod

4

O₂

118. A Hundred

10' easy warm up
2500m at 6k pace +8 @ 20 SPM, 10' rest
2500m at 6k pace +6 @ 22 SPM

39 min.

Mod

4

O₂

119. Step it Up

10' easy warm up
5' at 6k pace + 6 @ 20 SPM
4' at 6k pace + 6 @ 22 SPM
3' at 6k pace + 6 @ 24 SPM
2' at 6k pace + 6 @ 26 SPM
1' at 6k pace + 6 @ 28 SPM
2' at 6k pace + 6 @ 26 SPM
3' at 6k pace + 6 @ 24 SPM
4' at 6k pace + 6 @ 22 SPM
5' at 6k pace + 6 @ 20 SPM

120. Borealis

10' easy warm up
12' at 6k pace + 10 @ 23 SPM, 3' rest
12' at 6k pace + 6 @ 25 SPM, 3' rest
12' at 6k pace +2 @ 27 SPM

52 min.

Mod

4

O₂

MODERATE

121. Snooze Button

10' easy warm up
5' at 6k pace +15 @ 20 SPM
5' at 6k pace +12 @ 22 SPM
5' at 6k pace +10 @ 24 SPM
5' at 6k pace +8 @ 26 SPM
5' at 6k pace +6 @ 28 SPM

35 min.

Mod

4

O₂

122. Happy Dance

10' easy warm up
5' at 6k pace +6 @ 18 SPM
5' at 6k pace +6 @ 20 SPM
5' at 6k pace +6 @ 24 SPM
5' at 6k pace +6 @ 24 SPM

30 min.

Mod

4

O₂

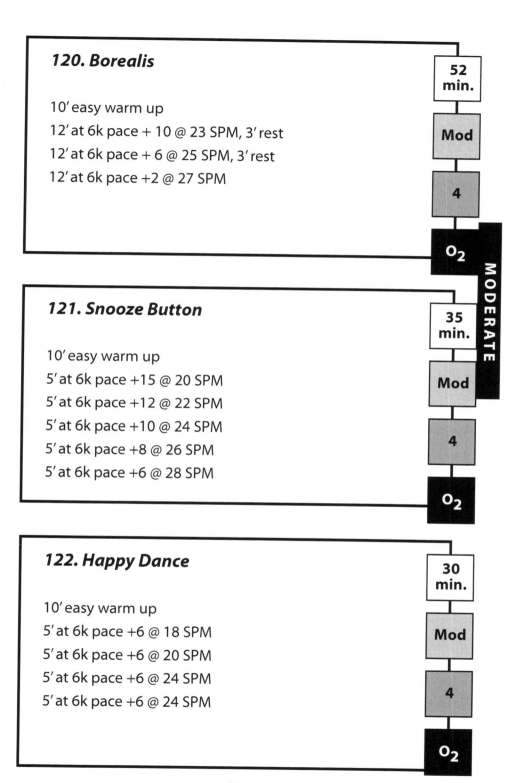

89

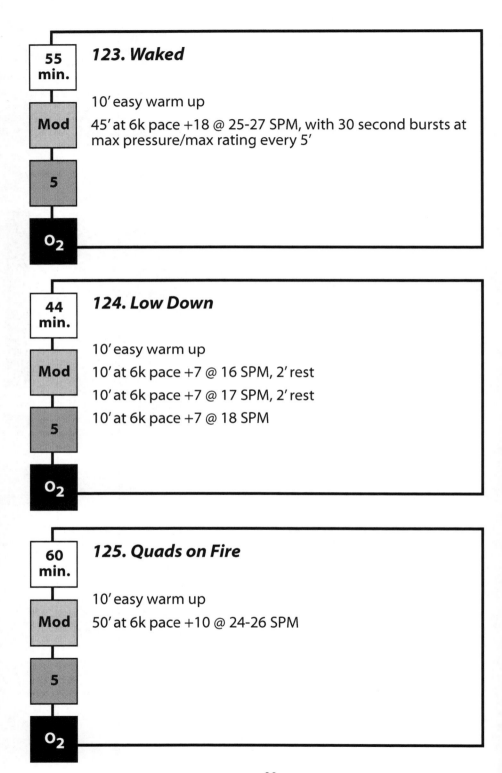

55 min.

Mod

5

O₂

123. Waked

10' easy warm up

45' at 6k pace +18 @ 25-27 SPM, with 30 second bursts at max pressure/max rating every 5'

44 min.

Mod

5

O₂

124. Low Down

10' easy warm up

10' at 6k pace +7 @ 16 SPM, 2' rest

10' at 6k pace +7 @ 17 SPM, 2' rest

10' at 6k pace +7 @ 18 SPM

60 min.

Mod

5

O₂

125. Quads on Fire

10' easy warm up

50' at 6k pace +10 @ 24-26 SPM

126. Ten and Twenties

10' easy warm up
20' at 6k pace +6 @ 22-24 SPM, 10' rest
20' at 6k pace +3 @ 24-26 SPM

60 min.

Mod

5

O₂

127. Ima Get You Sucka

10' easy warm up
1000m @ 18 SPM at 6k pace +10
1000m @ 20 SPM at 6k pace +8
1000m @ 22 SPM at 6k pace +6
1000m @ 24 SPM at 6k pace +4
1000m @ 22 SPM at 6k pace +6
1000m @ 20 SPM at 6k pace +8

45-65 min.

Mod

5

O₂

MODERATE

128. Slow Roll

10' easy warm up
8,000m at 75% pressure

75-90 min.

Mod

5

O₂

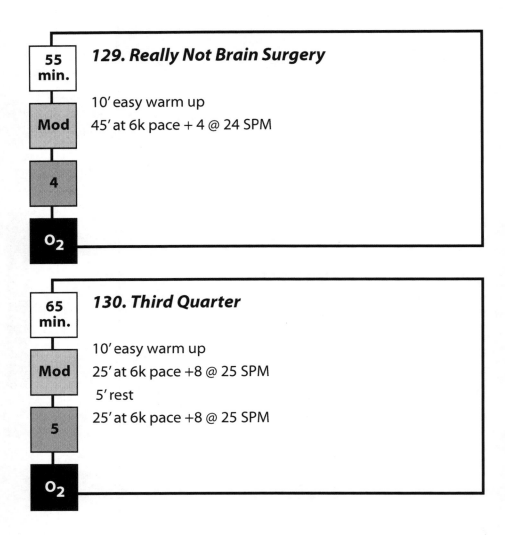

55 min.

Mod

4

O₂

129. Really Not Brain Surgery

10' easy warm up
45' at 6k pace + 4 @ 24 SPM

65 min.

Mod

5

O₂

130. Third Quarter

10' easy warm up
25' at 6k pace +8 @ 25 SPM
 5' rest
25' at 6k pace +8 @ 25 SPM

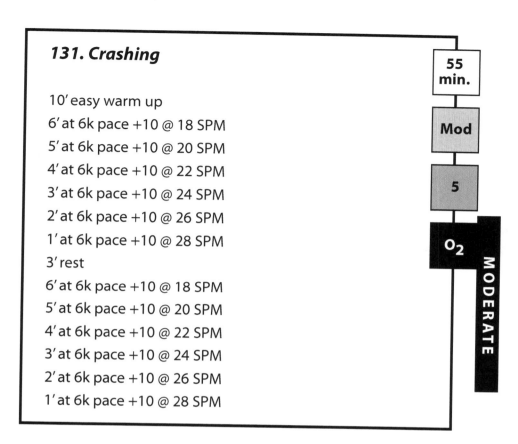

131. Crashing

55 min.

Mod

5

O₂

10' easy warm up
6' at 6k pace +10 @ 18 SPM
5' at 6k pace +10 @ 20 SPM
4' at 6k pace +10 @ 22 SPM
3' at 6k pace +10 @ 24 SPM
2' at 6k pace +10 @ 26 SPM
1' at 6k pace +10 @ 28 SPM
3' rest
6' at 6k pace +10 @ 18 SPM
5' at 6k pace +10 @ 20 SPM
4' at 6k pace +10 @ 22 SPM
3' at 6k pace +10 @ 24 SPM
2' at 6k pace +10 @ 26 SPM
1' at 6k pace +10 @ 28 SPM

MODERATE

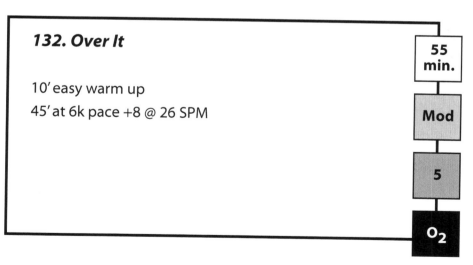

132. Over It

55 min.

Mod

5

O₂

10' easy warm up
45' at 6k pace +8 @ 26 SPM

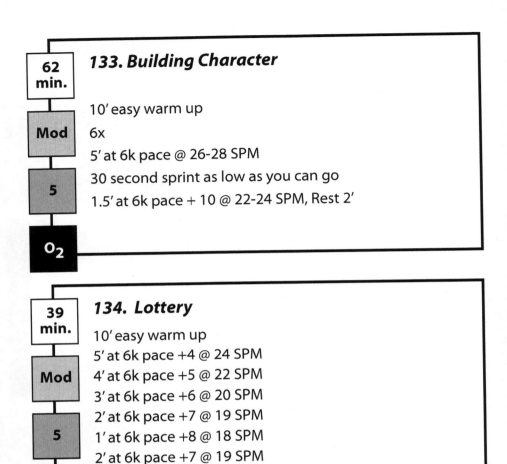

133. Building Character

62 min.

Mod

5

O₂

10' easy warm up
6x
5' at 6k pace @ 26-28 SPM
30 second sprint as low as you can go
1.5' at 6k pace + 10 @ 22-24 SPM, Rest 2'

134. Lottery

39 min.

Mod

5

O₂

10' easy warm up
5' at 6k pace +4 @ 24 SPM
4' at 6k pace +5 @ 22 SPM
3' at 6k pace +6 @ 20 SPM
2' at 6k pace +7 @ 19 SPM
1' at 6k pace +8 @ 18 SPM
2' at 6k pace +7 @ 19 SPM
3' at 6k pace +6 @ 20 SPM
4' at 6k pace +5 @ 22 SPM
5' at 6k pace +4 @ 24 SPM

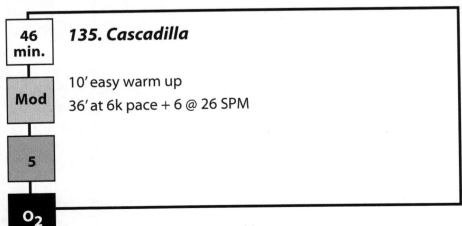

135. Cascadilla

46 min.

Mod

5

O₂

10' easy warm up
36' at 6k pace + 6 @ 26 SPM

136. Interest Rate

10' easy warm up

15' start at 6k pace + 10 @ 25 SPM, and drop your split by one each minute, finishing the piece at 6k pace -5

3' rest

15' start at 6k pace + 10 @ 25 SPM, and drop your split by one each minute, finishing the piece at 6k pace -5

43 min.

Mod

5

O₂

137. Opening Day

10' easy warm up

3x

10' at 6k pace + 6 @ 24 SPM

7' at 6k pace +6 @ 26 SPM

61 min.

MOD

5

O₂

MODERATE

138. Speed Bump

10' easy warm up

6000m at 6k pace +6 @ 18 SPM

30-60 min.

Mod

5

O₂

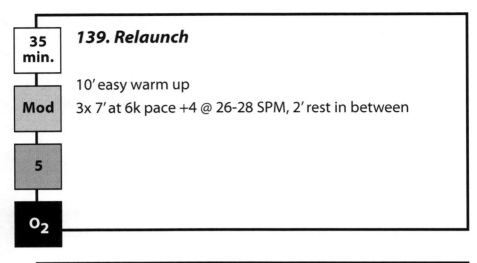

35 min.

Mod

5

O₂

139. Relaunch

10' easy warm up
3x 7' at 6k pace +4 @ 26-28 SPM, 2' rest in between

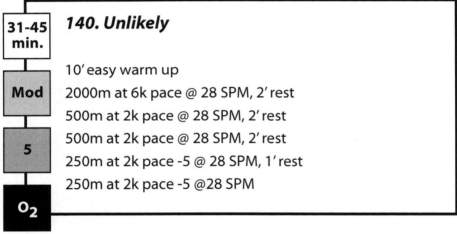

31-45 min.

Mod

5

O₂

140. Unlikely

10' easy warm up
2000m at 6k pace @ 28 SPM, 2' rest
500m at 2k pace @ 28 SPM, 2' rest
500m at 2k pace @ 28 SPM, 2' rest
250m at 2k pace -5 @ 28 SPM, 1' rest
250m at 2k pace -5 @28 SPM

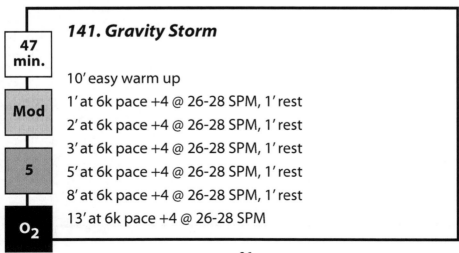

47 min.

Mod

5

O₂

141. Gravity Storm

10' easy warm up
1' at 6k pace +4 @ 26-28 SPM, 1' rest
2' at 6k pace +4 @ 26-28 SPM, 1' rest
3' at 6k pace +4 @ 26-28 SPM, 1' rest
5' at 6k pace +4 @ 26-28 SPM, 1' rest
8' at 6k pace +4 @ 26-28 SPM, 1' rest
13' at 6k pace +4 @ 26-28 SPM

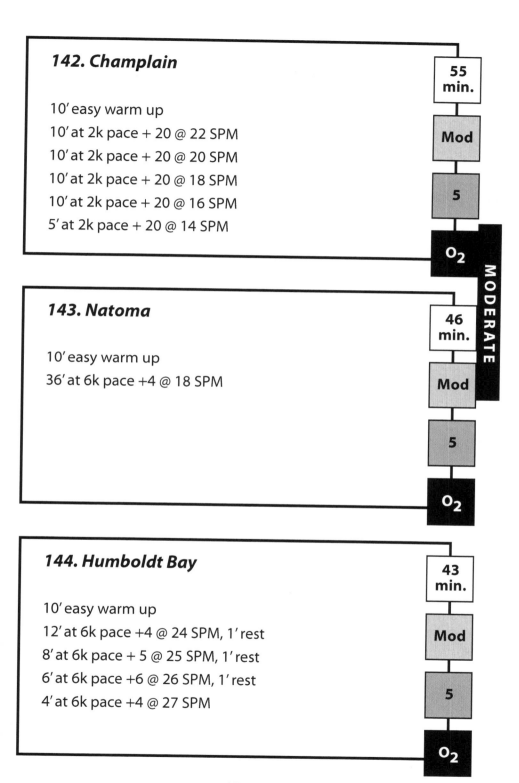

142. Champlain

10' easy warm up
10' at 2k pace + 20 @ 22 SPM
10' at 2k pace + 20 @ 20 SPM
10' at 2k pace + 20 @ 18 SPM
10' at 2k pace + 20 @ 16 SPM
5' at 2k pace + 20 @ 14 SPM

55 min.

Mod

5

O₂

143. Natoma

10' easy warm up
36' at 6k pace +4 @ 18 SPM

46 min.

Mod

5

O₂

MODERATE

144. Humboldt Bay

10' easy warm up
12' at 6k pace +4 @ 24 SPM, 1' rest
8' at 6k pace + 5 @ 25 SPM, 1' rest
6' at 6k pace +6 @ 26 SPM, 1' rest
4' at 6k pace +4 @ 27 SPM

43 min.

Mod

5

O₂

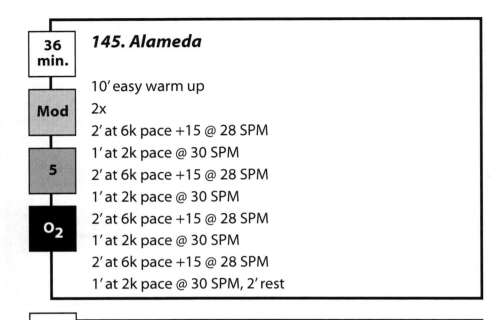

36 min.

Mod

5

O₂

145. Alameda

10' easy warm up
2x
2' at 6k pace +15 @ 28 SPM
1' at 2k pace @ 30 SPM
2' at 6k pace +15 @ 28 SPM
1' at 2k pace @ 30 SPM
2' at 6k pace +15 @ 28 SPM
1' at 2k pace @ 30 SPM
2' at 6k pace +15 @ 28 SPM
1' at 2k pace @ 30 SPM, 2' rest

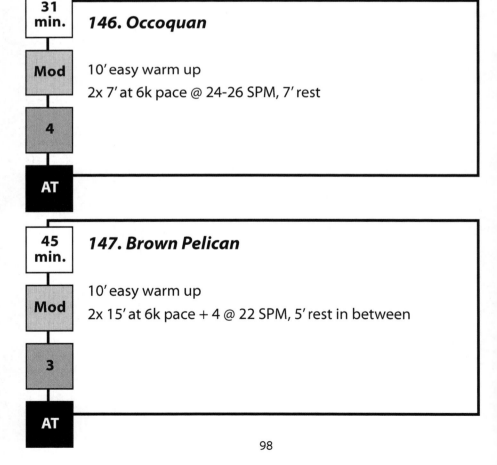

31 min.

Mod

4

AT

146. Occoquan

10' easy warm up
2x 7' at 6k pace @ 24-26 SPM, 7' rest

45 min.

Mod

3

AT

147. Brown Pelican

10' easy warm up
2x 15' at 6k pace + 4 @ 22 SPM, 5' rest in between

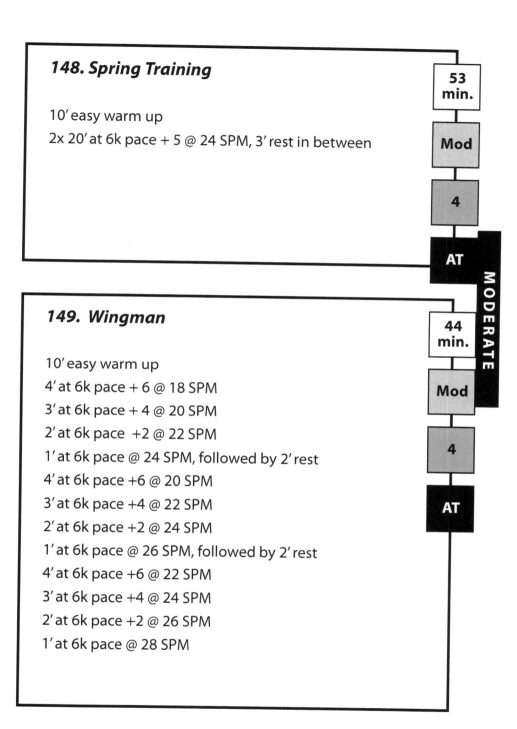

148. Spring Training

10' easy warm up
2x 20' at 6k pace + 5 @ 24 SPM, 3' rest in between

53 min.

Mod

4

AT

MODERATE

149. Wingman

10' easy warm up
4' at 6k pace + 6 @ 18 SPM
3' at 6k pace + 4 @ 20 SPM
2' at 6k pace +2 @ 22 SPM
1' at 6k pace @ 24 SPM, followed by 2' rest
4' at 6k pace +6 @ 20 SPM
3' at 6k pace +4 @ 22 SPM
2' at 6k pace +2 @ 24 SPM
1' at 6k pace @ 26 SPM, followed by 2' rest
4' at 6k pace +6 @ 22 SPM
3' at 6k pace +4 @ 24 SPM
2' at 6k pace +2 @ 26 SPM
1' at 6k pace @ 28 SPM

44 min.

Mod

4

AT

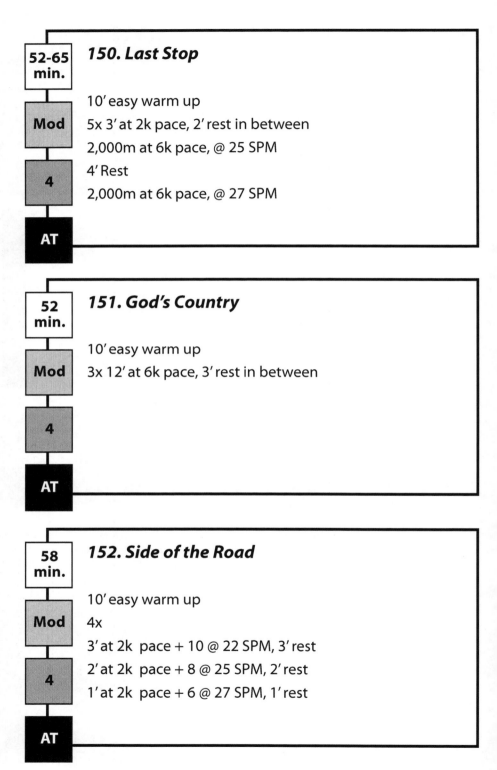

52-65 min.

Mod

4

AT

150. Last Stop

10' easy warm up
5x 3' at 2k pace, 2' rest in between
2,000m at 6k pace, @ 25 SPM
4' Rest
2,000m at 6k pace, @ 27 SPM

52 min.

Mod

4

AT

151. God's Country

10' easy warm up
3x 12' at 6k pace, 3' rest in between

58 min.

Mod

4

AT

152. Side of the Road

10' easy warm up
4x
3' at 2k pace + 10 @ 22 SPM, 3' rest
2' at 2k pace + 8 @ 25 SPM, 2' rest
1' at 2k pace + 6 @ 27 SPM, 1' rest

153. Superfly

10' easy warm up
6' at 2k pace +10 @ 20 SPM, 3' rest
5' at 2k pace +8 @ 22 SPM, 3' rest
4' at 2k pace +6 @ 24 SPM, 3' rest
3' at 2k pace +4 @ 26 SPM, 3' rest
2' at 2k pace +3 @ 28 SPM, 3' rest
1' at 2k pace @ 30 SPM

46 min.

Mod

4

AT

154. Hot Tar

10' easy warm up

6' at 6k pace +8 @ 20 SPM, 5' at 6k pace +8 @ 22 SPM,
4' at 6k pace +8 @ 24 SPM, 3' at 6k pace +8 @ 26 SPM,
2' at 6k pace +8 @ 28 SPM, 1' at 6k pace +8 @ 30 SPM

10' rest

6' at 6k pace +8 @ 20 SPM, 5' at 6k pace +8 @ 22 SPM,
4' at 6k pace +8 @ 24 SPM, 3' at 6k pace +8 @ 26 SPM,
2' at 6k pace +8 @ 28 SPM, 1' at 6k pace +8 @ 30 SPM

62 min.

Mod

4

AT

MODERATE

155. Criterion

10' easy warm up
3 x 6' at 2k pace +8 @ 26 SPM, 3' rest in between

34 min.

Mod

4

AT

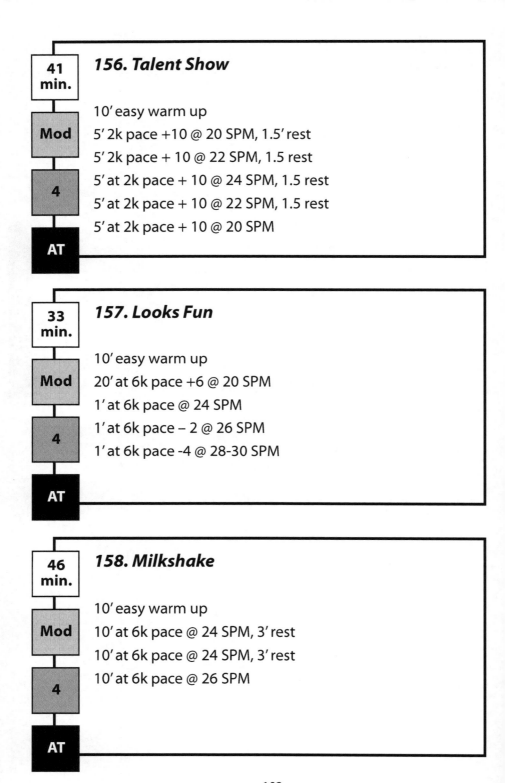

156. Talent Show

41 min.

Mod

4

AT

10' easy warm up
5' 2k pace +10 @ 20 SPM, 1.5' rest
5' 2k pace + 10 @ 22 SPM, 1.5 rest
5' at 2k pace + 10 @ 24 SPM, 1.5 rest
5' at 2k pace + 10 @ 22 SPM, 1.5 rest
5' at 2k pace + 10 @ 20 SPM

157. Looks Fun

33 min.

Mod

4

AT

10' easy warm up
20' at 6k pace +6 @ 20 SPM
1' at 6k pace @ 24 SPM
1' at 6k pace – 2 @ 26 SPM
1' at 6k pace -4 @ 28-30 SPM

158. Milkshake

46 min.

Mod

4

AT

10' easy warm up
10' at 6k pace @ 24 SPM, 3' rest
10' at 6k pace @ 24 SPM, 3' rest
10' at 6k pace @ 26 SPM

159. Lucky Penny

10' easy warm up
4x
1' at 6k pace @ 16 SPM
1' at 6k pace -1 @ 18 SPM
1' at 6k pace -2 @ 20 SPM
1' at 6k pace -3 @ 22 SPM
1' at 6k pace -4 @ 24 SPM
5' rest

45 min.

Mod

5

AT

160. Take Your Medicine

10' easy warm up
10' at 6k -2 @ 22 SPM, 2' rest
10' at 6k -3 @ 24 SPM, 2' rest
10' at 6k -4 @ 26 SPM

44 min.

Mod

5

AT

MODERATE

161. A Team

10' easy warm up
5x
0.5' at 2k pace @ 24 SPM, 0.5' rest
1' at 2k pace @ 26 SPM, 1' rest
1.5' at 2k pace @ 28 SPM, 1.5' rest
1' at 2k pace @ 26 SPM, 1' rest
0.5' at 2k pace @ 24 SPM, 0.5' rest

55 min.

Mod

5

AT

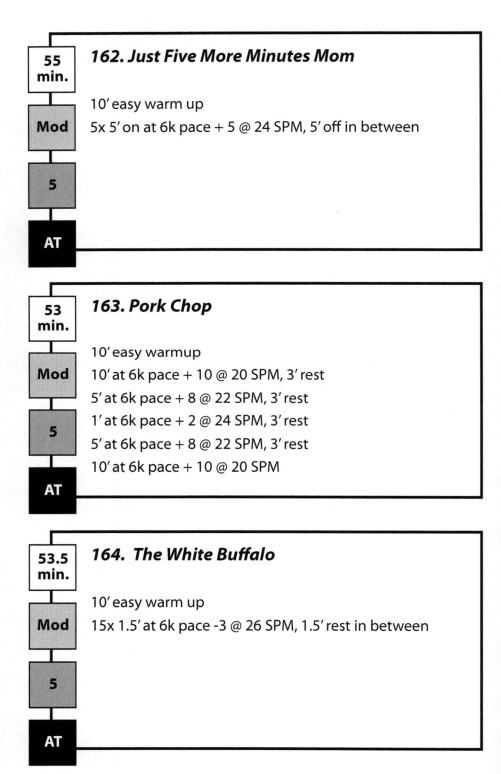

55 min.

Mod

5

AT

162. Just Five More Minutes Mom

10' easy warm up

5x 5' on at 6k pace + 5 @ 24 SPM, 5' off in between

53 min.

Mod

5

AT

163. Pork Chop

10' easy warmup

10' at 6k pace + 10 @ 20 SPM, 3' rest

5' at 6k pace + 8 @ 22 SPM, 3' rest

1' at 6k pace + 2 @ 24 SPM, 3' rest

5' at 6k pace + 8 @ 22 SPM, 3' rest

10' at 6k pace + 10 @ 20 SPM

53.5 min.

Mod

5

AT

164. The White Buffalo

10' easy warm up

15x 1.5' at 6k pace -3 @ 26 SPM, 1.5' rest in between

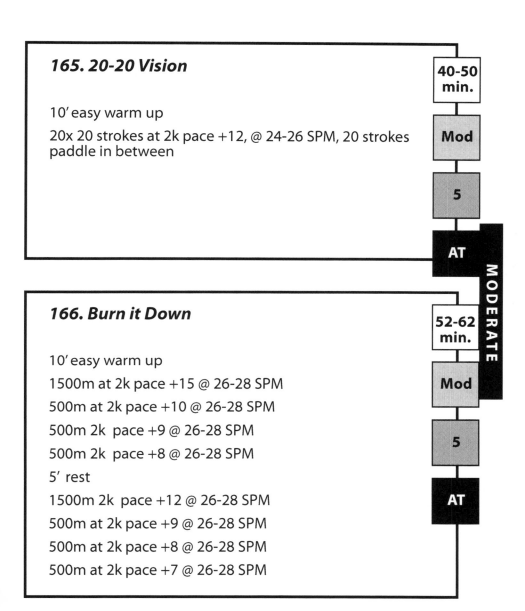

165. 20-20 Vision

10' easy warm up

20x 20 strokes at 2k pace +12, @ 24-26 SPM, 20 strokes paddle in between

40-50 min.

Mod

5

AT

166. Burn it Down

10' easy warm up

1500m at 2k pace +15 @ 26-28 SPM

500m at 2k pace +10 @ 26-28 SPM

500m 2k pace +9 @ 26-28 SPM

500m 2k pace +8 @ 26-28 SPM

5' rest

1500m 2k pace +12 @ 26-28 SPM

500m at 2k pace +9 @ 26-28 SPM

500m at 2k pace +8 @ 26-28 SPM

500m at 2k pace +7 @ 26-28 SPM

52-62 min.

Mod

5

AT

MODERATE

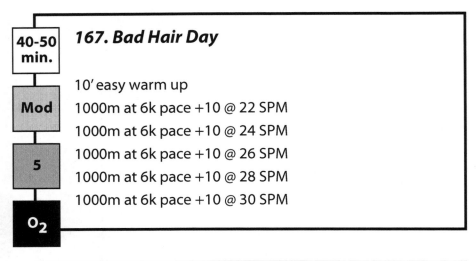

40-50 min.

Mod

5

O₂

167. Bad Hair Day

10' easy warm up
1000m at 6k pace +10 @ 22 SPM
1000m at 6k pace +10 @ 24 SPM
1000m at 6k pace +10 @ 26 SPM
1000m at 6k pace +10 @ 28 SPM
1000m at 6k pace +10 @ 30 SPM

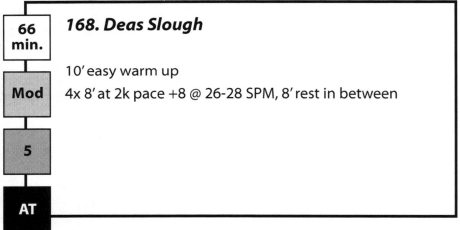

66 min.

Mod

5

AT

168. Deas Slough

10' easy warm up
4x 8' at 2k pace +8 @ 26-28 SPM, 8' rest in between

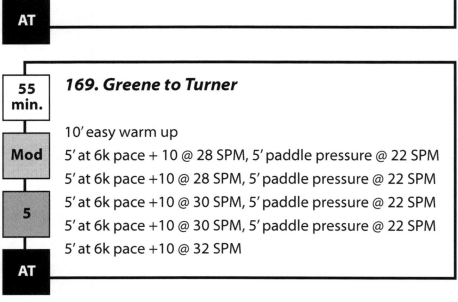

55 min.

Mod

5

AT

169. Greene to Turner

10' easy warm up
5' at 6k pace + 10 @ 28 SPM, 5' paddle pressure @ 22 SPM
5' at 6k pace +10 @ 28 SPM, 5' paddle pressure @ 22 SPM
5' at 6k pace +10 @ 30 SPM, 5' paddle pressure @ 22 SPM
5' at 6k pace +10 @ 30 SPM, 5' paddle pressure @ 22 SPM
5' at 6k pace +10 @ 32 SPM

170. Fremont Troll

30-40 min.

Mod

5

AT

10' easy warm up
1000m at 2k pace +12 @ 32 SPM, 3' rest
750m at 2k pace +10 @ 32 SPM, 2' rest
500m at 2k pace +8 @ 32 SPM, 1' rest
250m at max pressure @ max rating, 1' rest
250m at max pressure @ max rating

171. River Bend

37 min.

Mod

5

TR

10' easy warm up
7x 3' at 2k pace +8 @ 26 SPM, 1' rest in between

172. Extra Credit

33 min.

Mod

5

TR

10' easy warm up
2' at 2k pace +14 @ 24 SPM, 1' rest
2' at 2k pace +12 @ 26 SPM, 1' rest
2' at 2k pace +10 @ 28 SPM, 1' rest
2' at 2k pace +8 @ 30 SPM, 1' rest
2' at 2k pace +6 @ 32 SPM, 1' rest
2' at 2k pace +4 @ 34 SPM, 1' rest
2' at 2k pace +2 @ 36 SPM, 1' rest
2' at 2k pace @ 38 SPM

MODERATE

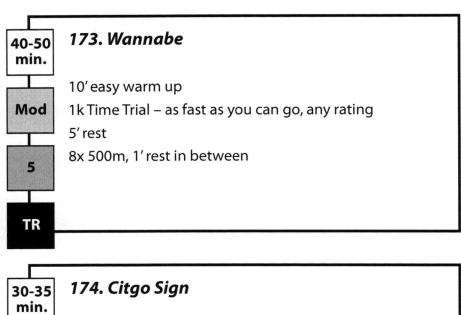

40-50 min.

Mod

5

TR

173. *Wannabe*

10' easy warm up
1k Time Trial – as fast as you can go, any rating
5' rest
8x 500m, 1' rest in between

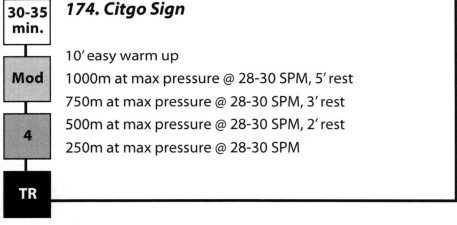

30-35 min.

Mod

4

TR

174. *Citgo Sign*

10' easy warm up
1000m at max pressure @ 28-30 SPM, 5' rest
750m at max pressure @ 28-30 SPM, 3' rest
500m at max pressure @ 28-30 SPM, 2' rest
250m at max pressure @ 28-30 SPM

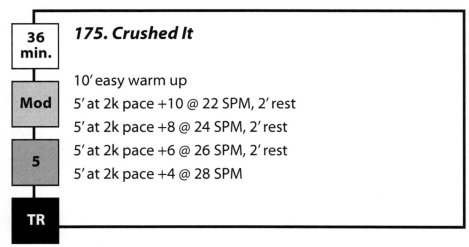

36 min.

Mod

5

TR

175. *Crushed It*

10' easy warm up
5' at 2k pace +10 @ 22 SPM, 2' rest
5' at 2k pace +8 @ 24 SPM, 2' rest
5' at 2k pace +6 @ 26 SPM, 2' rest
5' at 2k pace +4 @ 28 SPM

176. Berkeley High

10' easy warmup
5x 420m at 2k pace -4 @ max rate, 4:20' rest in between

38 min.

Mod

4

TR

MODERATE

177. Lucky Severn

10' easy warm up
15x 1' at 2k pace -2 @ 26 SPM, 1' rest in between

39 min.

Mod

5

TR

178. The Bends

10' easy warm up
5 x 3' at 2k pace -2 @ 24-26 SPM, 1' rest in between
5x 1.5' at 2k pace -3 @ 26-28 SPM, 0.5' rest in between

39.5 min.

Mod

5

TR

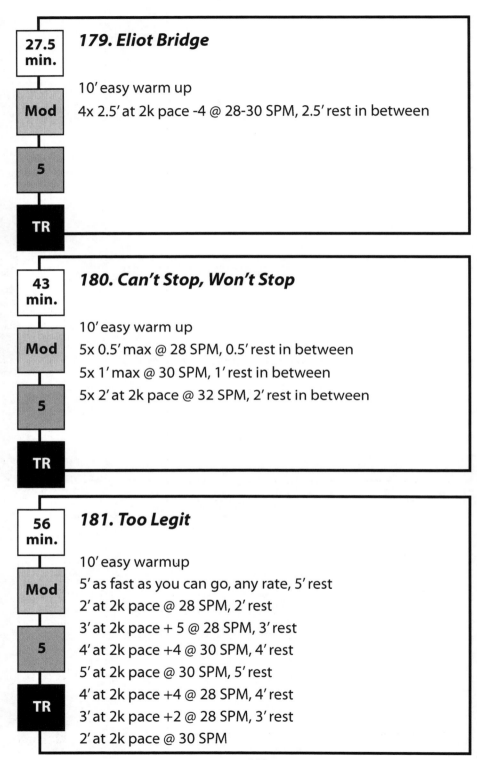

27.5 min.

Mod

5

TR

179. Eliot Bridge

10' easy warm up

4x 2.5' at 2k pace -4 @ 28-30 SPM, 2.5' rest in between

43 min.

Mod

5

TR

180. Can't Stop, Won't Stop

10' easy warm up

5x 0.5' max @ 28 SPM, 0.5' rest in between

5x 1' max @ 30 SPM, 1' rest in between

5x 2' at 2k pace @ 32 SPM, 2' rest in between

56 min.

Mod

5

TR

181. Too Legit

10' easy warmup

5' as fast as you can go, any rate, 5' rest

2' at 2k pace @ 28 SPM, 2' rest

3' at 2k pace + 5 @ 28 SPM, 3' rest

4' at 2k pace +4 @ 30 SPM, 4' rest

5' at 2k pace @ 30 SPM, 5' rest

4' at 2k pace +4 @ 28 SPM, 4' rest

3' at 2k pace +2 @ 28 SPM, 3' rest

2' at 2k pace @ 30 SPM

182. Not All Sunshine and Unicorns

10' easy warmup

10 x 650m at 2k pace -2, @ 28 SPM, with equal rest in between

50-65 min.

Mod

5

TR

MODERATE

183. The Hammer

10' easy warm up
4x 1' at 2k pace +2 @ 22 SPM, 1' rest
2' rest
4x 1' at 2k pace +2 @ 24 SPM, 1' rest
2' rest
4x 1' at 2k pace +2 @ 26 SPM, 1' rest
2' rest
4x 1' at 2k pace +2 @ 28 SPM, 1' rest

44 min.

Mod

5

TR

184. Stepping Up

10' easy warm up
3x
1' at 2k pace @ 24 SPM, 1' rest
2' at 2k pace @ 26 SPM, 2' rest
3' at 2k pace @ 28 SPM, 3' rest
2' at 2k pace @ 26 SPM, 2' rest
1' at 2k pace @ 24 SPM, 1' rest

63 min.

Mod

5

TR

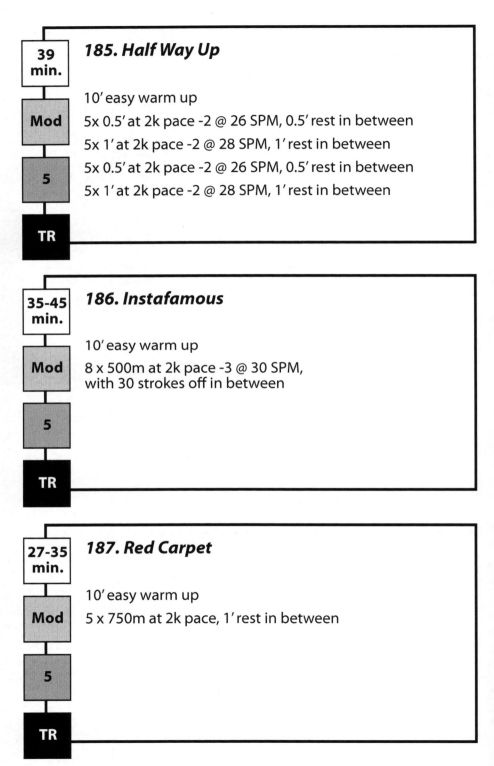

39 min.

Mod

5

TR

185. Half Way Up

10' easy warm up
5x 0.5' at 2k pace -2 @ 26 SPM, 0.5' rest in between
5x 1' at 2k pace -2 @ 28 SPM, 1' rest in between
5x 0.5' at 2k pace -2 @ 26 SPM, 0.5' rest in between
5x 1' at 2k pace -2 @ 28 SPM, 1' rest in between

35-45 min.

Mod

5

TR

186. Instafamous

10' easy warm up
8 x 500m at 2k pace -3 @ 30 SPM,
with 30 strokes off in between

27-35 min.

Mod

5

TR

187. Red Carpet

10' easy warm up
5 x 750m at 2k pace, 1' rest in between

188. Speeding Ticket

10' easy warm up
500m at 2k pace -1 @ 28 SPM, 2' rest
500m at 2k pace -2 @ 28 SPM, 2' rest
500m at 2k pace -3 @ 28 SPM, 2' rest
500m at 2k pace -4 @ 28 SPM, 2' rest
500m at 2k pace -5 @ 28 SPM, 2' rest
500m at 2k pace -6 @ 28 SPM, 2' rest
500m at 2k pace -7 @ 28 SPM

32-40 min.

Mod

5

TR

189. Fair Fight

10' easy warm up
1500m at 2k pace + 4 @ 26-28 SPM, 3' rest
5x 500m at 2k pace +4 @ 26-28 SPM, 1' rest in between
1500m at 2k pace +4 @ 26-28 SPM

35-42 min.

Mod

5

TR

MODERATE

190. Wolf Pack

10' easy warm up
5x 1200m at 2k pace +6 @ 28-30 SPM, 2' rest in between

40-50 min.

Mod

5

TR

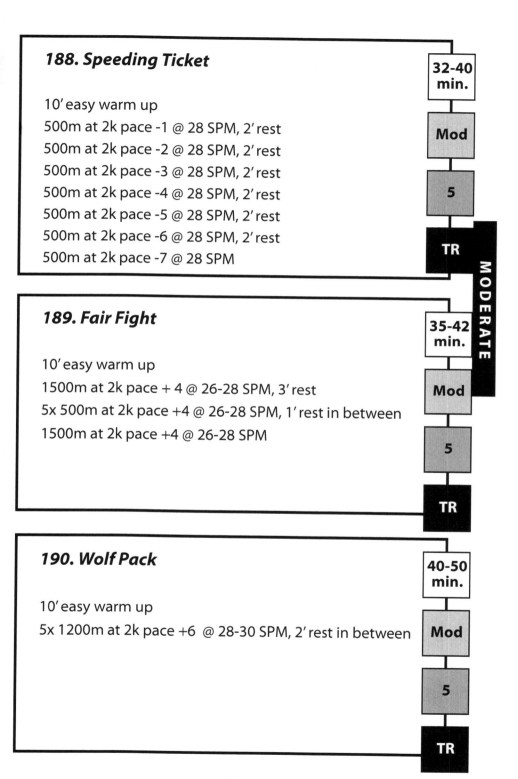

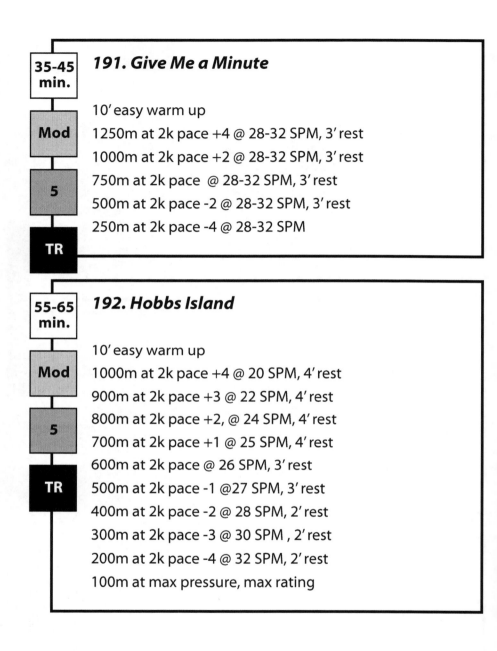

35-45 min.

Mod

5

TR

191. Give Me a Minute

10' easy warm up

1250m at 2k pace +4 @ 28-32 SPM, 3' rest

1000m at 2k pace +2 @ 28-32 SPM, 3' rest

750m at 2k pace @ 28-32 SPM, 3' rest

500m at 2k pace -2 @ 28-32 SPM, 3' rest

250m at 2k pace -4 @ 28-32 SPM

55-65 min.

Mod

5

TR

192. Hobbs Island

10' easy warm up

1000m at 2k pace +4 @ 20 SPM, 4' rest

900m at 2k pace +3 @ 22 SPM, 4' rest

800m at 2k pace +2, @ 24 SPM, 4' rest

700m at 2k pace +1 @ 25 SPM, 4' rest

600m at 2k pace @ 26 SPM, 3' rest

500m at 2k pace -1 @27 SPM, 3' rest

400m at 2k pace -2 @ 28 SPM, 2' rest

300m at 2k pace -3 @ 30 SPM , 2' rest

200m at 2k pace -4 @ 32 SPM, 2' rest

100m at max pressure, max rating

193. Fairmount

10' easy warm up
500m at 2k pace +2 @ 28 SPM, 1' rest
500m at 2k pace +1 @ 29 SPM, 1' rest
500m at 2k pace @ 30 SPM, 1' rest
500m at 2k pace -1 @ 31 SPM, 1' rest
500m at 2k pace -2 @ 32 SPM, 1' rest
500m at max pressure @ 33 SPM

26-30 min.

Mod

5

TR

194. Erie Canal

10' easy warm up
6x
2' at 2k pace -2 @ 26 SPM
1' at 2k pace -4 @ 28-30 SPM, 3' rest in between

43 min.

Mod

5

TR

MODERATE

195. Mendota

10' easy warm up
750m at 2k pace -4 @ 32-34 SPM
250m at max power @ 32-34 SPM
1000m at paddle pressure @ 20 SPM
750m at 2k pace -2 @ 32-34 SPM
250m at max power @ 32-34 SPM
1000m at paddle pressure @ 20 SPM
750m at 2k pace @ 32-34 SPM
250m at max power @ 32-34 SPM
1000m at paddle pressure @ 20 SPM

45-55 min.

Mod

5

TR

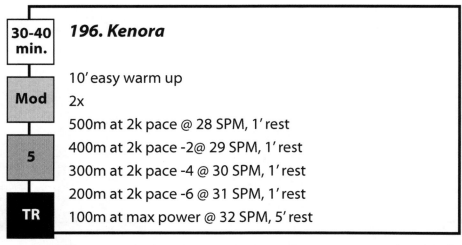

30-40 min.

Mod

5

TR

196. Kenora

10' easy warm up

2x

500m at 2k pace @ 28 SPM, 1' rest

400m at 2k pace -2 @ 29 SPM, 1' rest

300m at 2k pace -4 @ 30 SPM, 1' rest

200m at 2k pace -6 @ 31 SPM, 1' rest

100m at max power @ 32 SPM, 5' rest

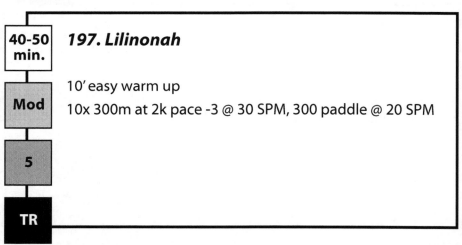

40-50 min.

Mod

5

TR

197. Lilinonah

10' easy warm up

10x 300m at 2k pace -3 @ 30 SPM, 300 paddle @ 20 SPM

ADVANCED WORKOUTS

When you're ready to put in some serious time and meters, you're ready for advanced workouts. We recommend doing all advanced erg workouts with what we call '10' easy warm up'. This includes rowing at 25% pressure for a first few minutes and steadily building to a light, comfortable, steady state rowing, no more than 75% of your max pressure. After the workout, spend at least 5 minutes on the erg in a light cool down.

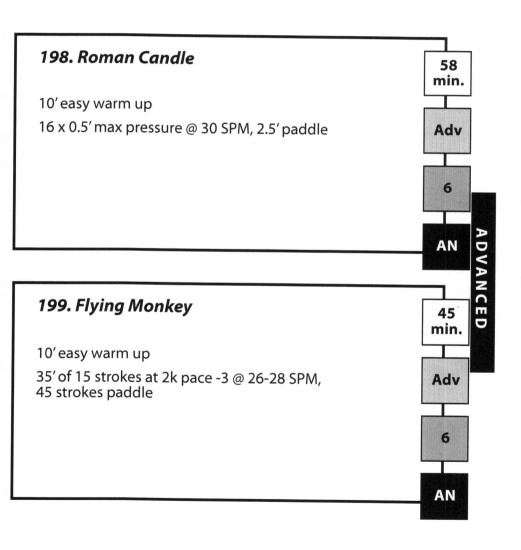

198. Roman Candle

10' easy warm up

16 x 0.5' max pressure @ 30 SPM, 2.5' paddle

58 min.

Adv

6

AN

199. Flying Monkey

10' easy warm up

35' of 15 strokes at 2k pace -3 @ 26-28 SPM, 45 strokes paddle

45 min.

Adv

6

AN

ADVANCED

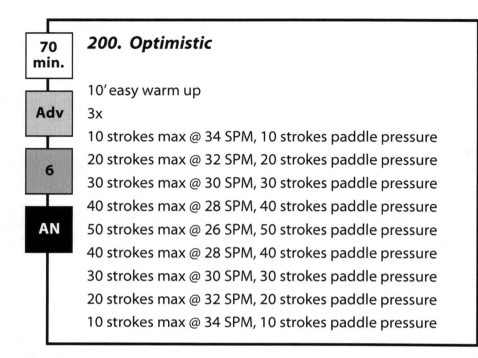

200. Optimistic

70 min.

Adv

6

AN

10' easy warm up

3x

10 strokes max @ 34 SPM, 10 strokes paddle pressure

20 strokes max @ 32 SPM, 20 strokes paddle pressure

30 strokes max @ 30 SPM, 30 strokes paddle pressure

40 strokes max @ 28 SPM, 40 strokes paddle pressure

50 strokes max @ 26 SPM, 50 strokes paddle pressure

40 strokes max @ 28 SPM, 40 strokes paddle pressure

30 strokes max @ 30 SPM, 30 strokes paddle pressure

20 strokes max @ 32 SPM, 20 strokes paddle pressure

10 strokes max @ 34 SPM, 10 strokes paddle pressure

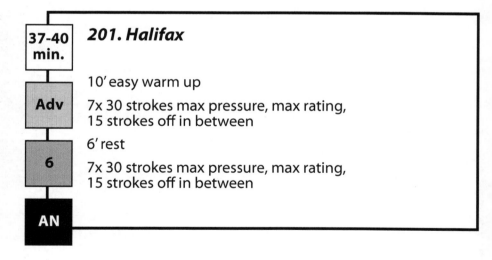

201. Halifax

37-40 min.

Adv

6

AN

10' easy warm up

7x 30 strokes max pressure, max rating,
15 strokes off in between

6' rest

7x 30 strokes max pressure, max rating,
15 strokes off in between

202. Carnegie Carnage

10' easy warm up

10x 1.5' at max power @ 30 SPM, 7.5' rest in between

92.5 min.

Adv

6

AN

203. The Rat

10' easy warm up

25x 0.5' at max power @ 30 SPM, 2.5' rest in between

82.5 min.

Adv

7

AN

ADVANCED

204. False Creek

10' easy warm up

4x

8x 20 sec at max power and max rating, 10 sec rest in between

10 min rest

110 min.

Adv

8

AN

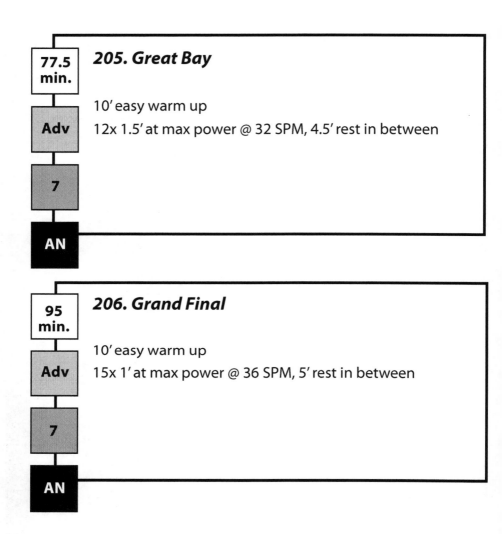

77.5 min.

Adv

7

AN

205. Great Bay

10' easy warm up

12x 1.5' at max power @ 32 SPM, 4.5' rest in between

95 min.

Adv

7

AN

206. Grand Final

10' easy warm up

15x 1' at max power @ 36 SPM, 5' rest in between

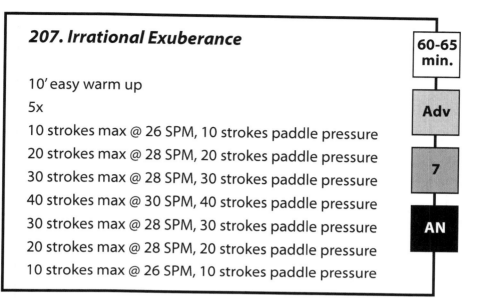

207. Irrational Exuberance

60-65 min.

Adv

7

AN

10' easy warm up

5x

10 strokes max @ 26 SPM, 10 strokes paddle pressure
20 strokes max @ 28 SPM, 20 strokes paddle pressure
30 strokes max @ 28 SPM, 30 strokes paddle pressure
40 strokes max @ 30 SPM, 40 strokes paddle pressure
30 strokes max @ 28 SPM, 30 strokes paddle pressure
20 strokes max @ 28 SPM, 20 strokes paddle pressure
10 strokes max @ 26 SPM, 10 strokes paddle pressure

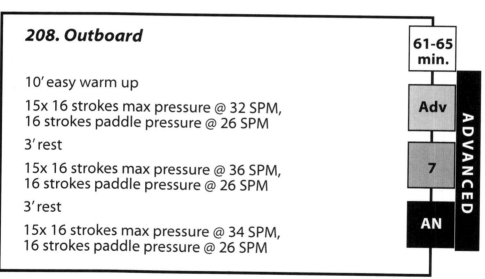

208. Outboard

61-65 min.

Adv

7

AN

ADVANCED

10' easy warm up

15x 16 strokes max pressure @ 32 SPM,
16 strokes paddle pressure @ 26 SPM

3' rest

15x 16 strokes max pressure @ 36 SPM,
16 strokes paddle pressure @ 26 SPM

3' rest

15x 16 strokes max pressure @ 34 SPM,
16 strokes paddle pressure @ 26 SPM

209. No Wake Zone

80.5 min.
Adv
8
AN

10' easy warm up
4x 1' at max pressure @ 32 SPM, 2' rest in between
5' rest
16x 0.5' max pressure @ 36 SPM, 0.5' rest in between
5' rest
4x 1' at max pressure @ 32 SPM, 2' rest in between
5' rest
16x 0.5' max pressure @ 34 SPM, 0.5' rest in between

210. What's Up?

60-65 min.
Adv
8
AN

10' easy warm up
20x 150m at 2k pace -5 @ 32 SPM, 150m off in between

211. Onota

81 min.
Adv
8
AN

10' easy warm up
15x 1' at max power @ 34-36 SPM, 4' rest in between

212. Picnic Point

10' easy warm up
10x 1.5' at max power @ 32 SPM, 6' rest in between

79 min.

Adv

8

AN

213. Mission Bay Mission

10' easy warm up
25x 0.5' at max power @ 36 SPM, 1.5' rest in between

58.5 min.

Adv

8

AN

ADVANCED

214. Serious Shade

20' at 75% pressure @ 22 SPM
12x 1' at max pressure/max rate, 4' rest in between

70-80 min.

Adv

6

AN

215. Third Level Final

50-60 min.

Adv

6

AN

20' at 75% pressure @ 22 SPM

4x 12 strokes at max pressure/max rate, 20 strokes paddle, 4' rest in between

216. DFL-abata

24 min.

Adv

6

AN

20' at 75% pressure @ 22 SPM

8x 20 seconds at max pressure/max rate, 10 seconds paddle

217. Totes M' Boats

40-45 min.

Adv

6

AN

20' at 75% pressure @ 22 SPM

4x 150m at max pressure/max rate, 2' rest in between

4' rest

4x 150m at max pressure/max rate, 2' rest in between

218. Lost and Found Sock

20' at 75% pressure @ 22 SPM

5x

10 seconds max pressure/max rate, 40 seconds off

20 seconds max pressure/max rate, 1' off

30 seconds max pressure/max rate, 2' off

15 seconds max pressure/max rate, 1' off

4' rest in between

62 min.

Adv

6

AN

219. Andiamo

20' at 75% pressure @ 22 SPM

6x 1.5' at max pressure/max rate, 4' rest in between

49 min.

Adv

6

AN

ADVANCED

220. The Goat

20' at 75% pressure @ 22-24 SPM

8x

100m at max pressure/max rate, 100m rest in between

30 min.

Adv

6

AN

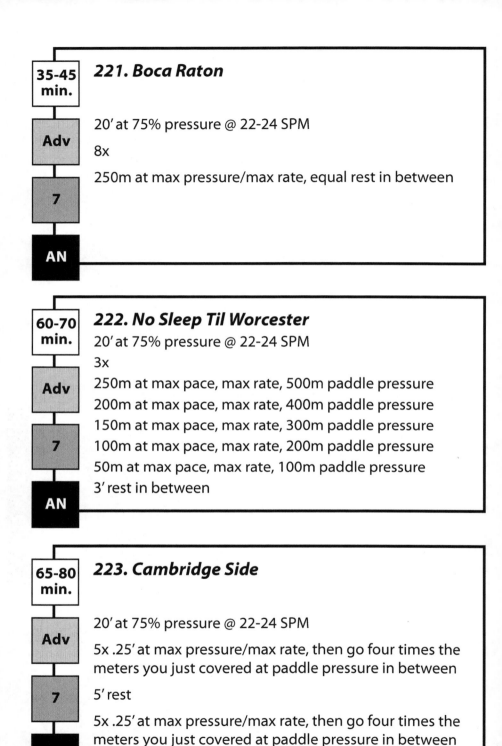

221. Boca Raton

35-45 min.

Adv

7

AN

20' at 75% pressure @ 22-24 SPM

8x

250m at max pressure/max rate, equal rest in between

222. No Sleep Til Worcester

60-70 min.

Adv

7

AN

20' at 75% pressure @ 22-24 SPM

3x

250m at max pace, max rate, 500m paddle pressure

200m at max pace, max rate, 400m paddle pressure

150m at max pace, max rate, 300m paddle pressure

100m at max pace, max rate, 200m paddle pressure

50m at max pace, max rate, 100m paddle pressure

3' rest in between

223. Cambridge Side

65-80 min.

Adv

7

AN

20' at 75% pressure @ 22-24 SPM

5x .25' at max pressure/max rate, then go four times the meters you just covered at paddle pressure in between

5' rest

5x .25' at max pressure/max rate, then go four times the meters you just covered at paddle pressure in between

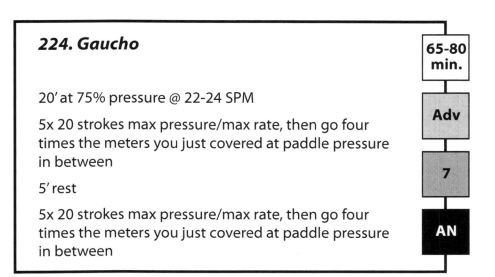

224. Gaucho

65-80 min.

Adv

7

AN

20' at 75% pressure @ 22-24 SPM

5x 20 strokes max pressure/max rate, then go four times the meters you just covered at paddle pressure in between

5' rest

5x 20 strokes max pressure/max rate, then go four times the meters you just covered at paddle pressure in between

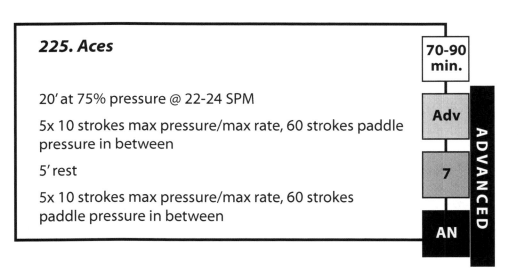

225. Aces

70-90 min.

Adv

7

AN

ADVANCED

20' at 75% pressure @ 22-24 SPM

5x 10 strokes max pressure/max rate, 60 strokes paddle pressure in between

5' rest

5x 10 strokes max pressure/max rate, 60 strokes paddle pressure in between

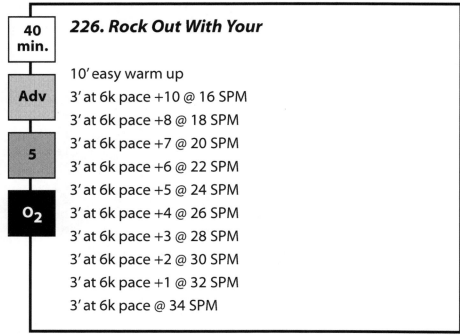

40 min.

Adv

5

O₂

226. Rock Out With Your

10' easy warm up

3' at 6k pace +10 @ 16 SPM

3' at 6k pace +8 @ 18 SPM

3' at 6k pace +7 @ 20 SPM

3' at 6k pace +6 @ 22 SPM

3' at 6k pace +5 @ 24 SPM

3' at 6k pace +4 @ 26 SPM

3' at 6k pace +3 @ 28 SPM

3' at 6k pace +2 @ 30 SPM

3' at 6k pace +1 @ 32 SPM

3' at 6k pace @ 34 SPM

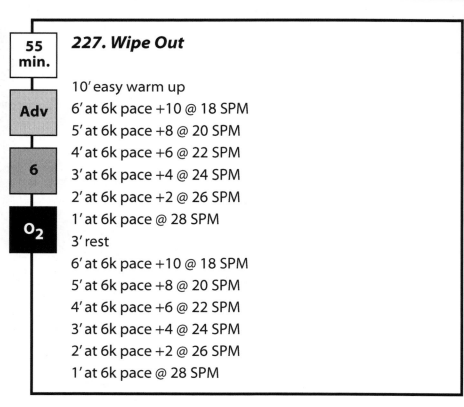

55 min.

Adv

6

O₂

227. Wipe Out

10' easy warm up

6' at 6k pace +10 @ 18 SPM

5' at 6k pace +8 @ 20 SPM

4' at 6k pace +6 @ 22 SPM

3' at 6k pace +4 @ 24 SPM

2' at 6k pace +2 @ 26 SPM

1' at 6k pace @ 28 SPM

3' rest

6' at 6k pace +10 @ 18 SPM

5' at 6k pace +8 @ 20 SPM

4' at 6k pace +6 @ 22 SPM

3' at 6k pace +4 @ 24 SPM

2' at 6k pace +2 @ 26 SPM

1' at 6k pace @ 28 SPM

228. Boxing Day

10' easy warm up
4' at 6k pace +5 @ 22 SPM
3' at 6k pace +4 @ 24 SPM
2' at 6k pace +3 @ 26 SPM
1' at 6k pace @ 28 SPM
Rest 3'
4' at 6k pace +5 @ 22 SPM
3' at 6k pace +4 @ 24 SPM
2' at 6k pace +3 @ 26 SPM
1' at 6k pace @ 28 SPM
Rest 3'
4' at 6k pace +5 @ 22 SPM
3' at 6k pace +4 @ 24 SPM
2' at 6k pace +3 @ 26 SPM
1' at 6k pace @ 28 SPM

46 min.

Adv

6

O₂

229. Velociraptor

10' easy warm up
10' at 6k pace @ 24 SPM
5x 0.5' at max @ 32 SPM, 0.5' at paddle @ 24 SPM in between
10' at 6k pace @ 24 SPM
5x 0.5' at max @ 32 SPM, 0.5' at paddle @ 24 SPM in between
10' at 6k pace @ 24 SPM

50 min.

Adv

6

O₂

ADVANCED

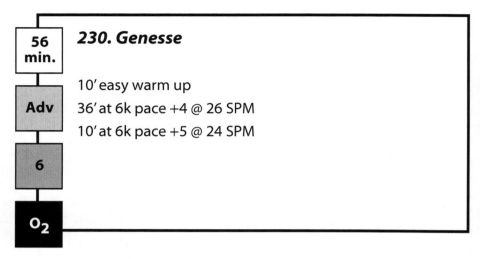

56 min.

Adv

6

O₂

230. Genesse

10' easy warm up
36' at 6k pace +4 @ 26 SPM
10' at 6k pace +5 @ 24 SPM

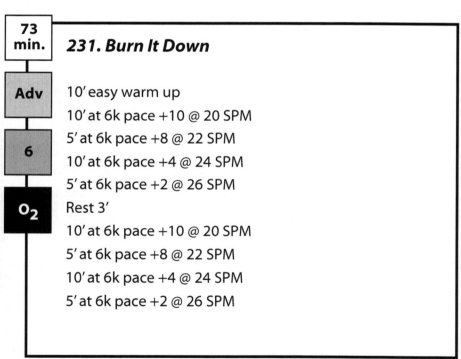

73 min.

Adv

6

O₂

231. Burn It Down

10' easy warm up
10' at 6k pace +10 @ 20 SPM
5' at 6k pace +8 @ 22 SPM
10' at 6k pace +4 @ 24 SPM
5' at 6k pace +2 @ 26 SPM
Rest 3'
10' at 6k pace +10 @ 20 SPM
5' at 6k pace +8 @ 22 SPM
10' at 6k pace +4 @ 24 SPM
5' at 6k pace +2 @ 26 SPM

232. Ready Steady

10' easy warm up
10' at 6k pace +13 @ 20 SPM
10' at 6k pace +11 @ 22 SPM
10' at 6k pace +9 @ 24 SPM
10' at 6k pace +7 @ 26 SPM
10' at 6k pace +5 @ 28 SPM

60 min.

Adv

6

O₂

233. Full Sail

10' easy warm up
5' at 6k pace +7 @ 18 SPM
5' at 6k pace +7 @ 20 SPM
5' at 6k pace +7 @ 22 SPM
5' at 6k pace +7 @ 24 SPM
5' at 6k pace +7 @ 26 SPM
5' at 6k pace +7 @ 28 SPM
5' at 6k pace +7 @ 30 SPM

45 min.

Adv

6

O₂

ADVANCED

234. Tornado Drill

10' easy warm up
32' at 6k pace @ 20 SPM
1' at 6k pace +6 @ 24 SPM
1' at 6k pace +4 @ 26 SPM
1' at 6k pace +2 @ 28-30 SPM

45 min.

Adv

6

O₂

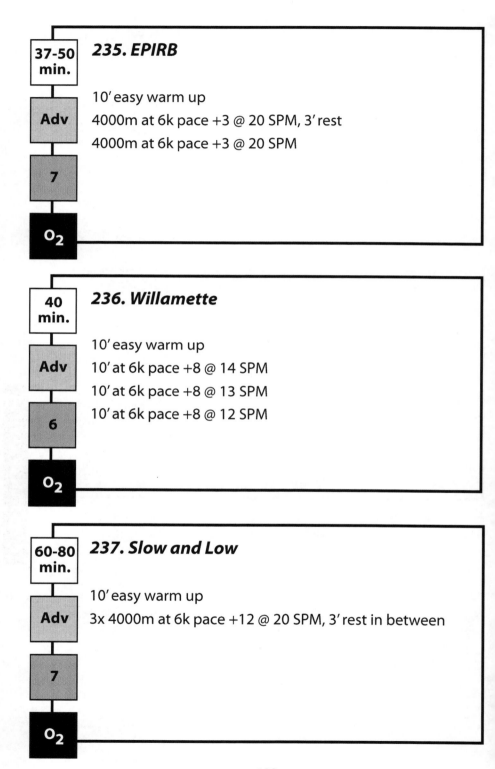

37-50 min.

Adv

7

O₂

235. EPIRB

10' easy warm up
4000m at 6k pace +3 @ 20 SPM, 3' rest
4000m at 6k pace +3 @ 20 SPM

40 min.

Adv

6

O₂

236. Willamette

10' easy warm up
10' at 6k pace +8 @ 14 SPM
10' at 6k pace +8 @ 13 SPM
10' at 6k pace +8 @ 12 SPM

60-80 min.

Adv

7

O₂

237. Slow and Low

10' easy warm up
3x 4000m at 6k pace +12 @ 20 SPM, 3' rest in between

238. Cliffhanger

10' easy warm up
6' at 6k pace +10 @ 18 SPM
5' at 6k pace +8 @ 20 SPM
4' at 6k pace +6 @ 22 SPM
3' at 6k pace +4 @ 24 SPM
2' at 6k pace +2 @ 26 SPM
1' at 6k pace @ 28 SPM
3' rest
6' at 6k pace +10 @ 18 SPM
5' at 6k pace +8 @ 20 SPM
4' at 6k pace +6 @ 22 SPM
3' at 6k pace +4 @ 24 SPM
2' at 6k pace +2 @ 26 SPM
1' at 6k pace @ 28 SPM
3' rest
6' at 6k pace +10 @ 18 SPM
5' at 6k pace +8 @ 20 SPM
4' at 6k pace +6 @ 22 SPM
3' at 6k pace +4 @ 24 SPM
2' at 6k pace +2 @ 26 SPM
1' at 6k pace @ 28 SPM

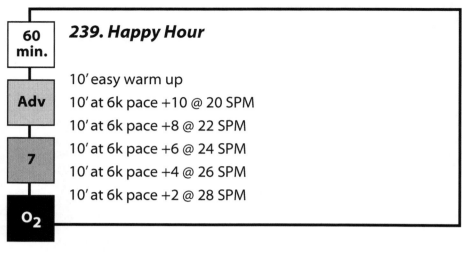

60 min.

Adv

7

O₂

239. Happy Hour

10' easy warm up
10' at 6k pace +10 @ 20 SPM
10' at 6k pace +8 @ 22 SPM
10' at 6k pace +6 @ 24 SPM
10' at 6k pace +4 @ 26 SPM
10' at 6k pace +2 @ 28 SPM

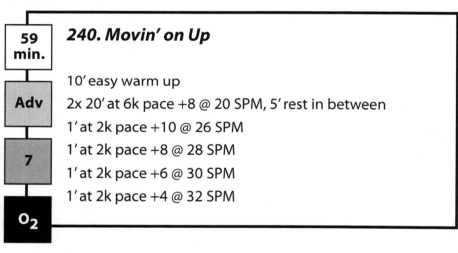

59 min.

Adv

7

O₂

240. Movin' on Up

10' easy warm up
2x 20' at 6k pace +8 @ 20 SPM, 5' rest in between
1' at 2k pace +10 @ 26 SPM
1' at 2k pace +8 @ 28 SPM
1' at 2k pace +6 @ 30 SPM
1' at 2k pace +4 @ 32 SPM

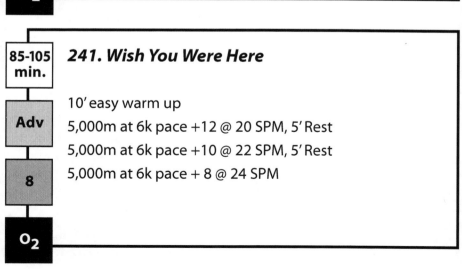

85-105 min.

Adv

8

O₂

241. Wish You Were Here

10' easy warm up
5,000m at 6k pace +12 @ 20 SPM, 5' Rest
5,000m at 6k pace +10 @ 22 SPM, 5' Rest
5,000m at 6k pace + 8 @ 24 SPM

242. Taste the Rainbow

10' easy warm up
10' at 6k pace +8 @ 20 SPM, 1' rest
10' at 6k pace +6 @ 22 SPM, 1' rest
10' at 6k pace +4 @ 24 SPM, 1' rest
10' at 6k pace +2 @ 26 SPM, 1' rest
10' at 6k pace @ 28 SPM

64 min.

Adv

7

O₂

243. Dirty Thirty

10' easy warm up
30' at 6k pace +6 @ 24 SPM
5' rest
30' at 6k pace +8 @ 24 SPM

75 min.

Adv

8

O₂

ADVANCED

244. Repachage

10' easy warm up
40' at 2k pace +15

50 min.

Adv

7

O₂

135

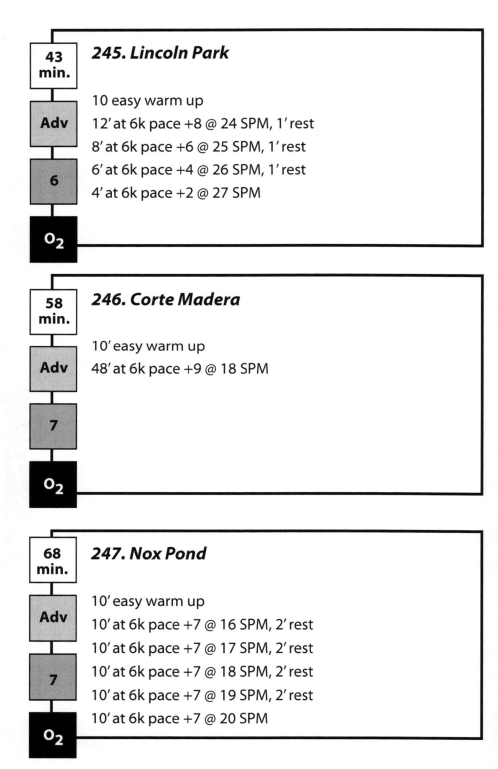

43 min.

Adv

6

O₂

245. Lincoln Park

10 easy warm up
12' at 6k pace +8 @ 24 SPM, 1' rest
8' at 6k pace +6 @ 25 SPM, 1' rest
6' at 6k pace +4 @ 26 SPM, 1' rest
4' at 6k pace +2 @ 27 SPM

58 min.

Adv

7

O₂

246. Corte Madera

10' easy warm up
48' at 6k pace +9 @ 18 SPM

68 min.

Adv

7

O₂

247. Nox Pond

10' easy warm up
10' at 6k pace +7 @ 16 SPM, 2' rest
10' at 6k pace +7 @ 17 SPM, 2' rest
10' at 6k pace +7 @ 18 SPM, 2' rest
10' at 6k pace +7 @ 19 SPM, 2' rest
10' at 6k pace +7 @ 20 SPM

248. Elk Lake

10' easy warm up
3x
10' at 6k pace -8 @ 24 SPM
7' at 6k pace -4 @ 26 SPM

61 min.

Adv

7

O₂

249. Dead Weight

10' easy warm up
10' at 2k pace +14 @ 22 SPM
10' at 2k pace +14 @ 20 SPM
10' at 2k pace +14 @ 18 SPM
10' at 2k pace +14 @ 16 SPM
5' at 2k pace +14 @ 14 SPM

55 min.

Adv

8

O₂

ADVANCED

250. Playing with Fire

10' easy warm up
3333m at 6k pace +6 @ 26-28 SPM, 5' rest
3333m at 6k pace +4 @ 26-28 SPM, sprint the last 250m

35-45 min.

Adv

8

O₂

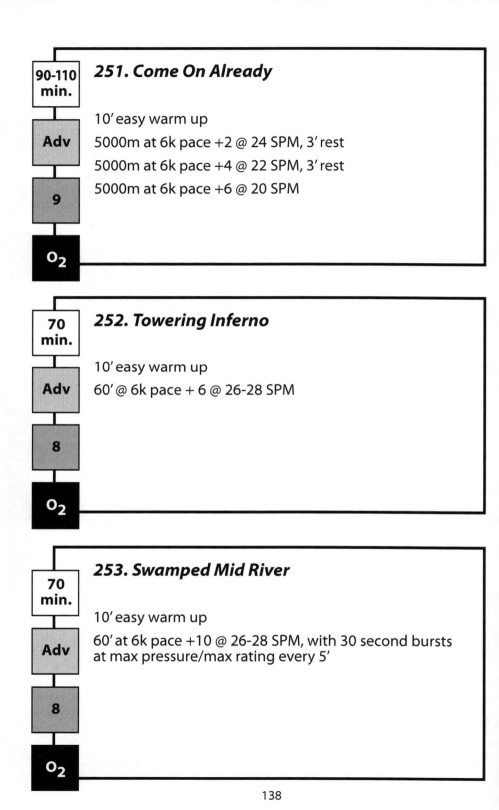

90-110 min.

Adv

9

O₂

251. Come On Already

10' easy warm up
5000m at 6k pace +2 @ 24 SPM, 3' rest
5000m at 6k pace +4 @ 22 SPM, 3' rest
5000m at 6k pace +6 @ 20 SPM

70 min.

Adv

8

O₂

252. Towering Inferno

10' easy warm up
60' @ 6k pace + 6 @ 26-28 SPM

70 min.

Adv

8

O₂

253. Swamped Mid River

10' easy warm up

60' at 6k pace +10 @ 26-28 SPM, with 30 second bursts at max pressure/max rating every 5'

254. Against the Law in Some Jurisdictions

| 90-120 min. |
| Adv |
| 10 |
| O₂ |

10,000m starting @ 16 SPM and increase rate every 2000m finishing @ 26 SPM

5' rest

2 x 20' at 6k pace +10 with 5' rest in between at any rating

255. 70 Plus

| 70 min. |
| Adv |
| 9 |
| O₂ |

10' easy warm up

60' at 6k pace +7 @ 28 SPM

256. Barrel of Monkeys

| 60 min. |
| Adv |
| 8 |
| O₂ |

10' easy warm up

10' at 6k pace +4 @ 24 SPM

10' at 6k pace +6 @ 26 SPM

10' at 6k pace +4 @ 28 SPM

10' at 6k pace +6 @ 26 SPM

10' at 6k pace +10 @ 24 SPM

ADVANCED

257. Nacho

85 min.

Adv

9

O₂

10' easy warm up
75' at 6k pace +12 @ 25 SPM

258. Monongahela

46-56 min.

Adv

7

O₂

10' easy warm up
6x 1500m at 2k pace +13 @ 28-30 SPM, 3' rest in between

259. Oak Ridge

60 min.

Adv

8

O₂

10' easy warm up
10' at 6k pace +8 @ 16 SPM
10' at 6k pace +8 @ 15 SPM
10' at 6k pace +8 @ 14 SPM
10' at 6k pace +8 @ 13 SPM
10' at 6k pace +8 @ 12 SPM

260. Hour of Power

10' easy warm up

60' as hard as you can go, rower's choice of rating

70 min.

Adv

9-10

O$_2$

261. Stick in the Eye

10' easy warm up

50' at 6k pace +8 @ 28-30 SPM, adding in power 10s every 5'

60 min.

Adv

9

O$_2$

ADVANCED

262. Straight Up Hour of Power

10' easy warm up

60' at 6k pace +6 @ 26-28 SPM

70 min.

Adv

9

O$_2$

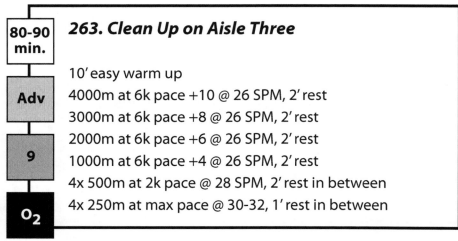

80-90 min.

Adv

9

O₂

263. Clean Up on Aisle Three

10' easy warm up
4000m at 6k pace +10 @ 26 SPM, 2' rest
3000m at 6k pace +8 @ 26 SPM, 2' rest
2000m at 6k pace +6 @ 26 SPM, 2' rest
1000m at 6k pace +4 @ 26 SPM, 2' rest
4x 500m at 2k pace @ 28 SPM, 2' rest in between
4x 250m at max pace @ 30-32, 1' rest in between

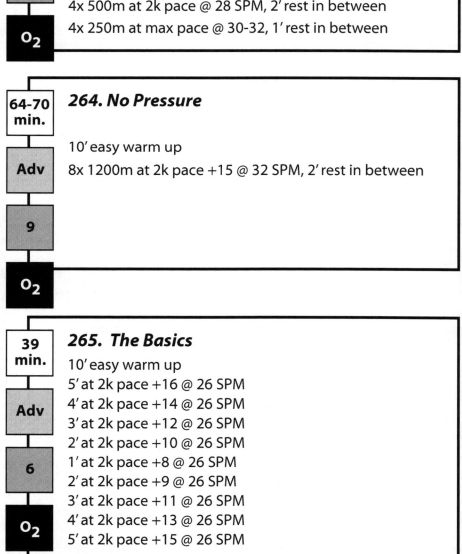

64-70 min.

Adv

9

O₂

264. No Pressure

10' easy warm up
8x 1200m at 2k pace +15 @ 32 SPM, 2' rest in between

39 min.

Adv

6

O₂

265. The Basics

10' easy warm up
5' at 2k pace +16 @ 26 SPM
4' at 2k pace +14 @ 26 SPM
3' at 2k pace +12 @ 26 SPM
2' at 2k pace +10 @ 26 SPM
1' at 2k pace +8 @ 26 SPM
2' at 2k pace +9 @ 26 SPM
3' at 2k pace +11 @ 26 SPM
4' at 2k pace +13 @ 26 SPM
5' at 2k pace +15 @ 26 SPM

266. Off the Rails

10' easy warm up
40' at 6k pace +8 @ 26 SPM
5' rest
40' at 6k pace +6 @ 26 SPM

95 min.

Adv

9

O₂

267. Grrranimals

10' easy warm up
3x
1500m at 2k pace +15 @ 20 SPM
500m at 2k pace +10 @ 22 SPM
500m at 2k pace +8 @ 24 SPM
500m at 2k pace +6 @ 26 SPM
500m at 2k pace +4 @ 28 SPM

50-70 min.

Adv

9

O₂

ADVANCED

268. Drip Sweat

10' easy warm up
3x 6000m at 6k pace + 10 @ 25-27 SPM, 5' rest in between

100-130 min.

Adv

9

O₂

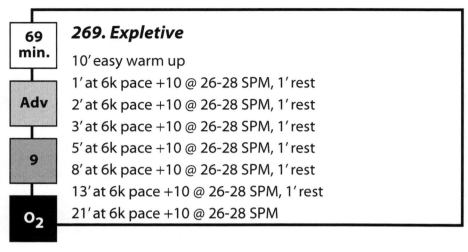

69 min.

Adv

9

O₂

269. Expletive

10' easy warm up

1' at 6k pace +10 @ 26-28 SPM, 1' rest

2' at 6k pace +10 @ 26-28 SPM, 1' rest

3' at 6k pace +10 @ 26-28 SPM, 1' rest

5' at 6k pace +10 @ 26-28 SPM, 1' rest

8' at 6k pace +10 @ 26-28 SPM, 1' rest

13' at 6k pace +10 @ 26-28 SPM, 1' rest

21' at 6k pace +10 @ 26-28 SPM

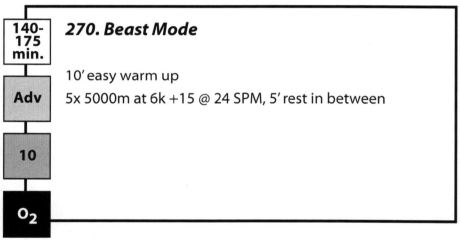

140-175 min.

Adv

10

O₂

270. Beast Mode

10' easy warm up

5x 5000m at 6k +15 @ 24 SPM, 5' rest in between

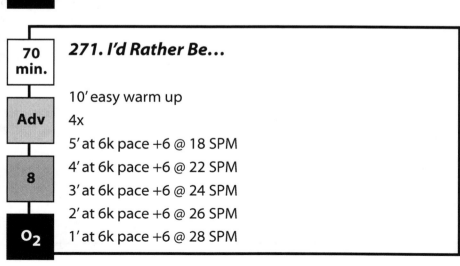

70 min.

Adv

8

O₂

271. I'd Rather Be...

10' easy warm up

4x

5' at 6k pace +6 @ 18 SPM

4' at 6k pace +6 @ 22 SPM

3' at 6k pace +6 @ 24 SPM

2' at 6k pace +6 @ 26 SPM

1' at 6k pace +6 @ 28 SPM

272. Longest Day

90-150 min.

Adv

9

O₂

10' easy warm up
10,000m at 6k pace +13 @ 26 SPM, 4' rest
10,000m at 6k pace +16 @ 26 SPM

273. Ghost Erg

60-70 min.

Adv

9

O₂

10' easy warm up
2000m at 6k pace +6 @ 28-32 SPM, 5' rest
2000m at 6k pace +12 @ 26-28 SPM, 5' rest
2000m at 6k pace +12 @ 26-28 SPM, 5' rest
2000m at 6k pace +6 @ 28-32 SPM

ADVANCED

274. U Lake 131

131 min

Adv

10

O₂

32' at 6k pace +15 @ 22-26 SPM, 1' rest
16' at 6k pace +15 @ 22-26 SPM, 1' rest
8' at 6k pace +15 @ 22-26 SPM, 1' rest
4' at 6k pace +15 @ 22-26 SPM, 6' rest
4' at 6k pace +15 @ 22-26 SPM, 1' rest
8' at 6k pace +15 @ 22-26 SPM, 1' rest
16' at 6k pace +15 @ 22-26 SPM, 1' rest
32' at 6k pace +15 @ 22-26 SPM

275. Lever Lung

70 min.

Adv

9

O₂

10' easy warm up
60' of 60 strokes on at 2k pace +15 @ 22-26 SPM, 1' off

276. Sixty Minute Trial

60 min.

Adv

10

O₂

60' as fast as you can go, for as many meters as you can go

277. The Real Half Marathon

75-110 min.

Adv

10

O₂

10' easy warm up
21,097m as fast as possible, at any rate

278. Marathon Trial

10' easy warm up
42,195m as fast as you can, at any rate

2.5-3.5 hrs.

Adv

10

O₂

279. I Woke Up Like This

10' easy warm up
10x 5' at 6k pace @ 24 SPM with 5' rest in between

105 min.

Adv

7

AT

ADVANCED

280. Throwback

10' easy warm up
3000m at 6k pace -2 @ 22 SPM, 2' rest
3000m at 6k pace -3 @ 24 SPM, 2' rest
3000m at 6k pace -4 @ 26 SPM

55-70 min.

Adv

7

AT

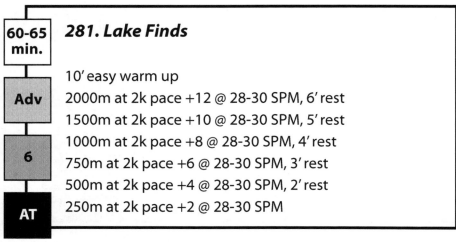

60-65 min.

Adv

6

AT

281. Lake Finds

10' easy warm up
2000m at 2k pace +12 @ 28-30 SPM, 6' rest
1500m at 2k pace +10 @ 28-30 SPM, 5' rest
1000m at 2k pace +8 @ 28-30 SPM, 4' rest
750m at 2k pace +6 @ 28-30 SPM, 3' rest
500m at 2k pace +4 @ 28-30 SPM, 2' rest
250m at 2k pace +2 @ 28-30 SPM

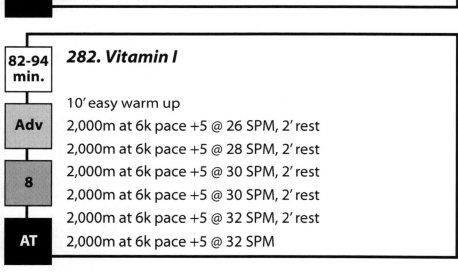

82-94 min.

Adv

8

AT

282. Vitamin I

10' easy warm up
2,000m at 6k pace +5 @ 26 SPM, 2' rest
2,000m at 6k pace +5 @ 28 SPM, 2' rest
2,000m at 6k pace +5 @ 30 SPM, 2' rest
2,000m at 6k pace +5 @ 30 SPM, 2' rest
2,000m at 6k pace +5 @ 32 SPM, 2' rest
2,000m at 6k pace +5 @ 32 SPM

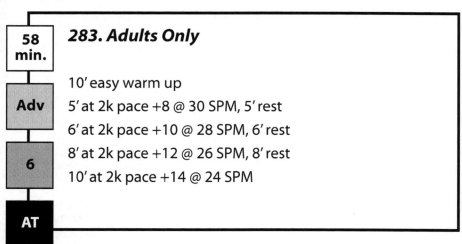

58 min.

Adv

6

AT

283. Adults Only

10' easy warm up
5' at 2k pace +8 @ 30 SPM, 5' rest
6' at 2k pace +10 @ 28 SPM, 6' rest
8' at 2k pace +12 @ 26 SPM, 8' rest
10' at 2k pace +14 @ 24 SPM

284. Citation

10' easy warm up
5x 6' at 2k pace +9 @ 26-28 SPM, 3' rest in between

| 52 min. |
| Adv |
| 6 |
| AT |

285. High Tide

10' easy warm up
4x 1500m at 2k pace +9 @ 28 SPM, 4' rest in between

| 45-48 min. |
| Adv |
| 6 |
| AT |

ADVANCED

286. Every Little Bit

10' easy warm up
5x
4' at 6k pace +4 @ 28 SPM
1' at 6k pace @ 30-32 SPM
5' rest in between

| 55 min. |
| Mod |
| 6 |
| AT |

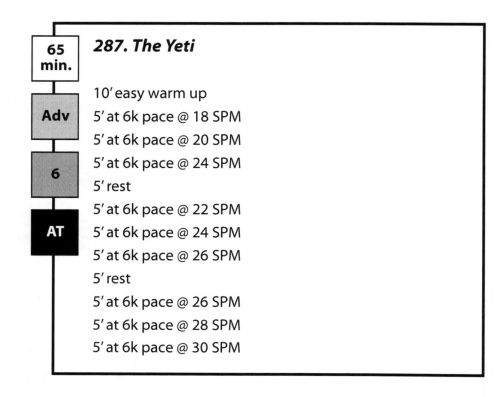

65 min.

Adv

6

AT

287. The Yeti

10' easy warm up
5' at 6k pace @ 18 SPM
5' at 6k pace @ 20 SPM
5' at 6k pace @ 24 SPM
5' rest
5' at 6k pace @ 22 SPM
5' at 6k pace @ 24 SPM
5' at 6k pace @ 26 SPM
5' rest
5' at 6k pace @ 26 SPM
5' at 6k pace @ 28 SPM
5' at 6k pace @ 30 SPM

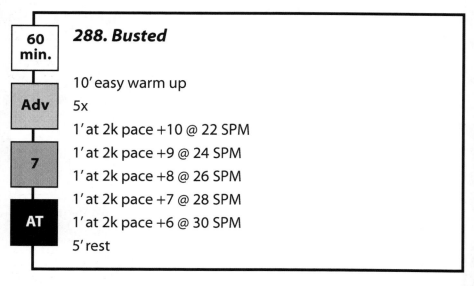

60 min.

Adv

7

AT

288. Busted

10' easy warm up
5x
1' at 2k pace +10 @ 22 SPM
1' at 2k pace +9 @ 24 SPM
1' at 2k pace +8 @ 26 SPM
1' at 2k pace +7 @ 28 SPM
1' at 2k pace +6 @ 30 SPM
5' rest

289. Creepin'

10' easy warm up
2000m at 6k pace +2 @ 22 SPM, 3' rest
3000m at 6k pace +4 @ 24 SPM, 3' rest
4000m at 6k pace +6 @ 26 SPM

50-70 min.

Adv

7

AT

290. The Rosen Bomb

10' easy warm up
5x 0.5' at 2k pace +10 @ 24 SPM, 0.5' rest
5x 1' at 2k pace +11 @ 26 SPM, 1' rest
5x 1.5' at 2k pace +12 @ 28 SPM, 1.5' rest
5x 2' at 2k pace +13 @ 28 SPM, 2' rest
5x 1.5' at 2k pace +12 @ 28 SPM, 1.5' rest
5x 1' at 2k pace +11 @ 26 SPM, 1' rest
5x 0.5' at 2k pace +10 @ 24 SPM, 0.5' rest

90 min.

Adv

7

AT

ADVANCED

291. 'A' Mountain Brush Fire

10' easy warm up
6x 5' at 2k pace +10 @ 30 SPM, 5' rest in between

65 min.

Adv

7

AT

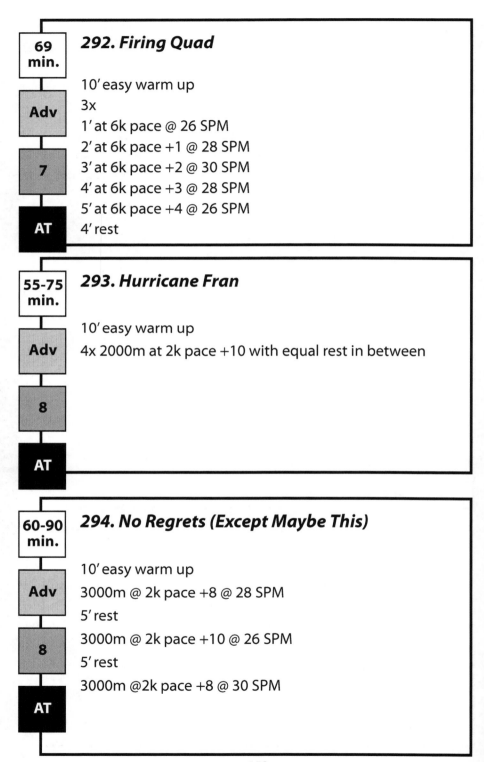

69 min.

Adv

7

AT

292. Firing Quad

10' easy warm up
3x
1' at 6k pace @ 26 SPM
2' at 6k pace +1 @ 28 SPM
3' at 6k pace +2 @ 30 SPM
4' at 6k pace +3 @ 28 SPM
5' at 6k pace +4 @ 26 SPM
4' rest

55-75 min.

Adv

8

AT

293. Hurricane Fran

10' easy warm up
4x 2000m at 2k pace +10 with equal rest in between

60-90 min.

Adv

8

AT

294. No Regrets (Except Maybe This)

10' easy warm up
3000m @ 2k pace +8 @ 28 SPM
5' rest
3000m @ 2k pace +10 @ 26 SPM
5' rest
3000m @2k pace +8 @ 30 SPM

295. Sweet Sixteen

65-90 min.

Adv

8

AT

10' easy warm up
4000m at 6k pace +6 @ 22 SPM, 2' rest
4000m at 6k pace +4 @ 24 SPM, 2' rest
4000m at 6k pace +2 @ 26 SPM

296. Weird Vibe

27 min.

Adv

6

AT

10' easy warm up
1' at 2k pace +12 @ 16 SPM
1' at 2k pace +12 @ 18 SPM
1' at 2k pace +12 @ 20 SPM
1' at 2k pace +12 @ 22 SPM
1' at 2k pace +12 @ 24 SPM
1' at 2k pace +12 @ 26 SPM
1' at 2k pace +12 @ 28 SPM
1' at 2k pace +12 @ 30 SPM
1' rest
1' at 2k pace +8 @ 16 SPM
1' at 2k pace +8 @ 18 SPM
1' at 2k pace +8 @ 20 SPM
1' at 2k pace +8 @ 22 SPM
1' at 2k pace +8 @ 24 SPM
1' at 2k pace +8 @ 26 SPM
1' at 2k pace +8 @ 28 SPM
1' at 2k pace +8 @ 30 SPM

ADVANCED

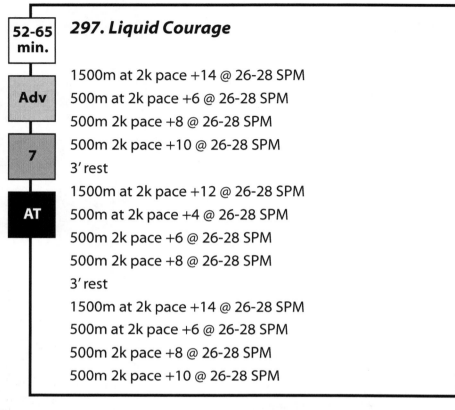

52-65 min.

Adv

7

AT

297. Liquid Courage

1500m at 2k pace +14 @ 26-28 SPM

500m at 2k pace +6 @ 26-28 SPM

500m 2k pace +8 @ 26-28 SPM

500m 2k pace +10 @ 26-28 SPM

3' rest

1500m at 2k pace +12 @ 26-28 SPM

500m at 2k pace +4 @ 26-28 SPM

500m 2k pace +6 @ 26-28 SPM

500m 2k pace +8 @ 26-28 SPM

3' rest

1500m at 2k pace +14 @ 26-28 SPM

500m at 2k pace +6 @ 26-28 SPM

500m 2k pace +8 @ 26-28 SPM

500m 2k pace +10 @ 26-28 SPM

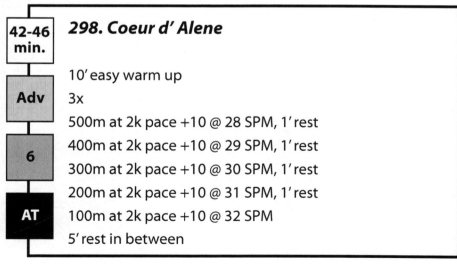

42-46 min.

Adv

6

AT

298. Coeur d' Alene

10' easy warm up

3x

500m at 2k pace +10 @ 28 SPM, 1' rest

400m at 2k pace +10 @ 29 SPM, 1' rest

300m at 2k pace +10 @ 30 SPM, 1' rest

200m at 2k pace +10 @ 31 SPM, 1' rest

100m at 2k pace +10 @ 32 SPM

5' rest in between

299. It's Complicated

82 min.

Adv

8

AT

10' easy warm up
2' @ 6k pace +1, @ 26 SPM, 2' rest
4' @ 6k pace +1, @ 26 SPM, 4' rest
6' @ 6k pace +1, @ 26 SPM, 6' rest
8' @ 6k pace +1, @ 26 SPM, 8' rest
7' @ 6k pace +1, @ 26 SPM, 7' rest
5' @ 6k pace +1, @ 26 SPM, 5' rest
3' @ 6k pace +1, @ 26 SPM, 3' rest
1' @ 6k pace +1, @ 26 SPM

300. For Days

90-120 min.

Adv

9

AT

10' easy warm up
6000m at 6k pace +6 @ 24 SPM, 5' rest
6000m at 6k pace +4 @ 26 SPM, 5' rest
6000m at 6k pace +6 @ 24 SPM

ADVANCED

301. Revolutionary

43-48 min.

Adv

8

AT

10' easy warm up
1000m at 2k pace +10 @ 32 SPM, 4' rest
750m at 2k pace +8 @ 32 SPM, 3' rest
500m at 2k pace +6 @ 32 SPM, 3' rest
250m at max pressure @ max rating, 2' rest
750 at 2k pace +6 @ 32 SPM

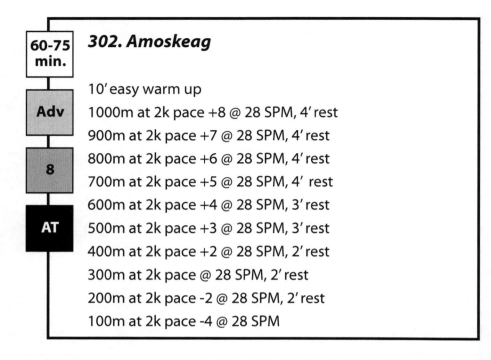

60-75 min.

Adv

8

AT

302. Amoskeag

10' easy warm up
1000m at 2k pace +8 @ 28 SPM, 4' rest
900m at 2k pace +7 @ 28 SPM, 4' rest
800m at 2k pace +6 @ 28 SPM, 4' rest
700m at 2k pace +5 @ 28 SPM, 4' rest
600m at 2k pace +4 @ 28 SPM, 3' rest
500m at 2k pace +3 @ 28 SPM, 3' rest
400m at 2k pace +2 @ 28 SPM, 2' rest
300m at 2k pace @ 28 SPM, 2' rest
200m at 2k pace -2 @ 28 SPM, 2' rest
100m at 2k pace -4 @ 28 SPM

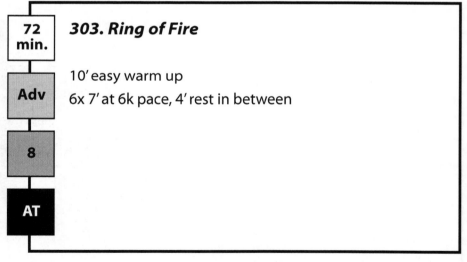

72 min.

Adv

8

AT

303. Ring of Fire

10' easy warm up
6x 7' at 6k pace, 4' rest in between

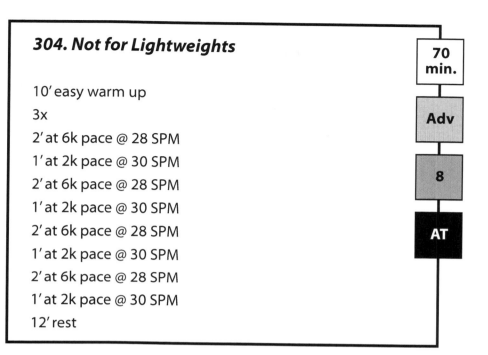

304. Not for Lightweights

70 min.

Adv

8

AT

10' easy warm up
3x
2' at 6k pace @ 28 SPM
1' at 2k pace @ 30 SPM
2' at 6k pace @ 28 SPM
1' at 2k pace @ 30 SPM
2' at 6k pace @ 28 SPM
1' at 2k pace @ 30 SPM
2' at 6k pace @ 28 SPM
1' at 2k pace @ 30 SPM
12' rest

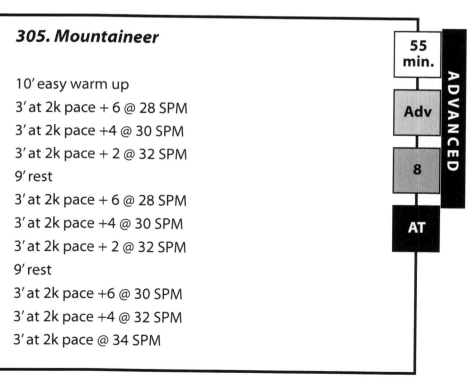

305. Mountaineer

55 min.

Adv

8

AT

ADVANCED

10' easy warm up
3' at 2k pace + 6 @ 28 SPM
3' at 2k pace +4 @ 30 SPM
3' at 2k pace + 2 @ 32 SPM
9' rest
3' at 2k pace + 6 @ 28 SPM
3' at 2k pace +4 @ 30 SPM
3' at 2k pace + 2 @ 32 SPM
9' rest
3' at 2k pace +6 @ 30 SPM
3' at 2k pace +4 @ 32 SPM
3' at 2k pace @ 34 SPM

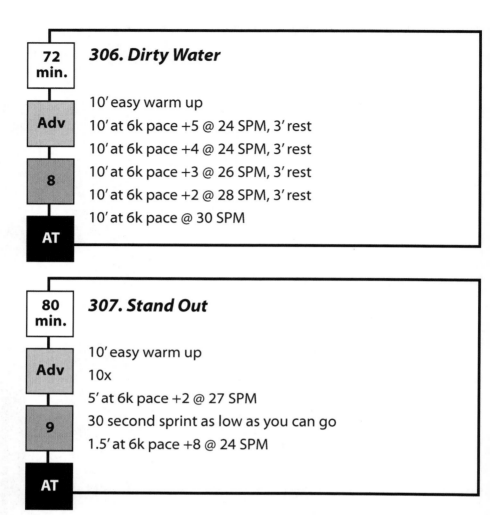

72 min.

Adv

8

AT

306. Dirty Water

10' easy warm up
10' at 6k pace +5 @ 24 SPM, 3' rest
10' at 6k pace +4 @ 24 SPM, 3' rest
10' at 6k pace +3 @ 26 SPM, 3' rest
10' at 6k pace +2 @ 28 SPM, 3' rest
10' at 6k pace @ 30 SPM

80 min.

Adv

9

AT

307. Stand Out

10' easy warm up
10x
5' at 6k pace +2 @ 27 SPM
30 second sprint as low as you can go
1.5' at 6k pace +8 @ 24 SPM

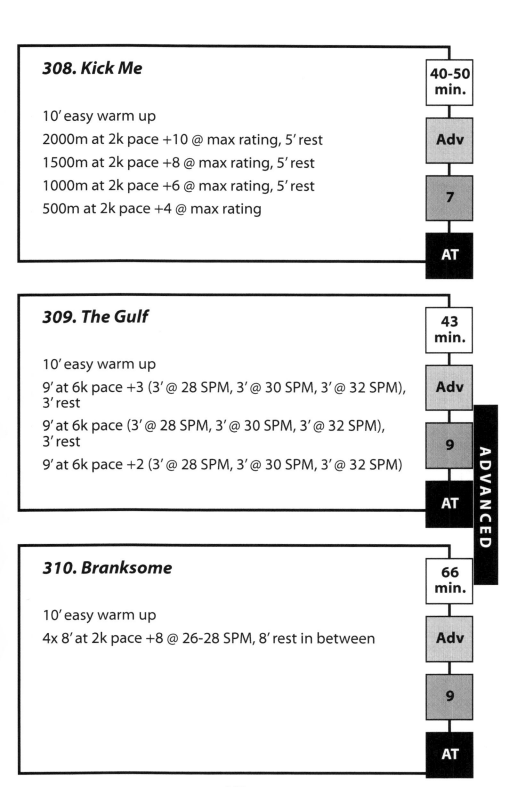

308. Kick Me

10' easy warm up

2000m at 2k pace +10 @ max rating, 5' rest

1500m at 2k pace +8 @ max rating, 5' rest

1000m at 2k pace +6 @ max rating, 5' rest

500m at 2k pace +4 @ max rating

40-50 min.

Adv

7

AT

309. The Gulf

10' easy warm up

9' at 6k pace +3 (3' @ 28 SPM, 3' @ 30 SPM, 3' @ 32 SPM), 3' rest

9' at 6k pace (3' @ 28 SPM, 3' @ 30 SPM, 3' @ 32 SPM), 3' rest

9' at 6k pace +2 (3' @ 28 SPM, 3' @ 30 SPM, 3' @ 32 SPM)

43 min.

Adv

9

AT

ADVANCED

310. Branksome

10' easy warm up

4x 8' at 2k pace +8 @ 26-28 SPM, 8' rest in between

66 min.

Adv

9

AT

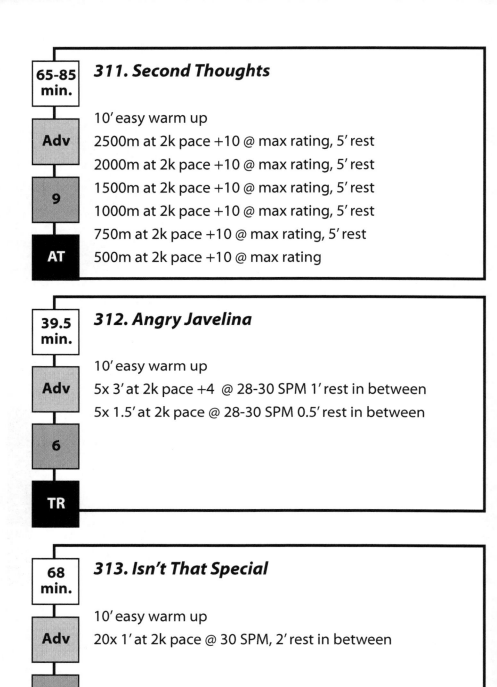

65-85 min.

Adv

9

AT

311. Second Thoughts

10' easy warm up
2500m at 2k pace +10 @ max rating, 5' rest
2000m at 2k pace +10 @ max rating, 5' rest
1500m at 2k pace +10 @ max rating, 5' rest
1000m at 2k pace +10 @ max rating, 5' rest
750m at 2k pace +10 @ max rating, 5' rest
500m at 2k pace +10 @ max rating

39.5 min.

Adv

6

TR

312. Angry Javelina

10' easy warm up
5x 3' at 2k pace +4 @ 28-30 SPM 1' rest in between
5x 1.5' at 2k pace @ 28-30 SPM 0.5' rest in between

68 min.

Adv

8

TR

313. Isn't That Special

10' easy warm up
20x 1' at 2k pace @ 30 SPM, 2' rest in between

314. Pi

10' easy warm up

15x 2' at 2k pace -2 @ 28-32 SPM, 2' rest in between

68 min.

Adv

7

TR

315. Not All Sunshine and Unicorns

10' easy warm up

10x 650m at 2k pace -2 @ 28 SPM, with equal rest in between

60-70 min.

Adv

6

TR

ADVANCED

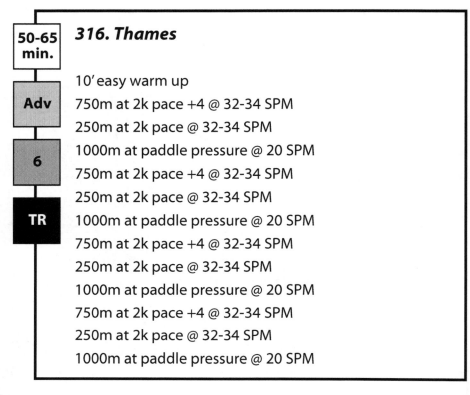

50-65 min.

Adv

6

TR

316. Thames

10' easy warm up
750m at 2k pace +4 @ 32-34 SPM
250m at 2k pace @ 32-34 SPM
1000m at paddle pressure @ 20 SPM
750m at 2k pace +4 @ 32-34 SPM
250m at 2k pace @ 32-34 SPM
1000m at paddle pressure @ 20 SPM
750m at 2k pace +4 @ 32-34 SPM
250m at 2k pace @ 32-34 SPM
1000m at paddle pressure @ 20 SPM
750m at 2k pace +4 @ 32-34 SPM
250m at 2k pace @ 32-34 SPM
1000m at paddle pressure @ 20 SPM

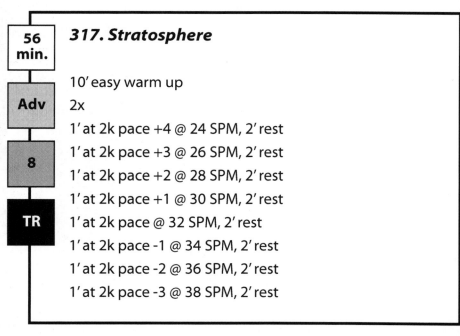

56 min.

Adv

8

TR

317. Stratosphere

10' easy warm up
2x
1' at 2k pace +4 @ 24 SPM, 2' rest
1' at 2k pace +3 @ 26 SPM, 2' rest
1' at 2k pace +2 @ 28 SPM, 2' rest
1' at 2k pace +1 @ 30 SPM, 2' rest
1' at 2k pace @ 32 SPM, 2' rest
1' at 2k pace -1 @ 34 SPM, 2' rest
1' at 2k pace -2 @ 36 SPM, 2' rest
1' at 2k pace -3 @ 38 SPM, 2' rest

318. Brown Cloud

10' easy warm up

10x alternating 40 strokes at 2k pace +4 @ 26 SPM, 10 strokes paddle

5' rest

10x alternating 40 strokes at 2k pace @ 30 SPM, 10 strokes paddle

5' rest

10x alternating 40 strokes at 2k pace +4 @ 26 SPM, 10 strokes paddle

75-95 min.

Adv

6

TR

319. El Camino

10' easy warm up

45' of 10 strokes at 2k pace +4 @ 24 SPM, 10 strokes at 2k pace +2 @ 26 SPM, 10 strokes at 2k pace @ 28 SPM, 30 strokes off

55 min.

Adv

6

TR

ADVANCED

320. Thank You, Easter Bunny

10' easy warm up

6x 5' @ 2k pace +4, 5' rest in between

65 min.

Adv

6

TR

163

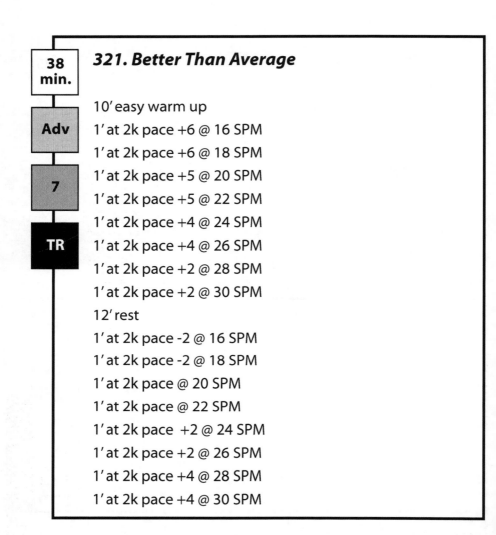

38 min.

Adv

7

TR

321. Better Than Average

10' easy warm up
1' at 2k pace +6 @ 16 SPM
1' at 2k pace +6 @ 18 SPM
1' at 2k pace +5 @ 20 SPM
1' at 2k pace +5 @ 22 SPM
1' at 2k pace +4 @ 24 SPM
1' at 2k pace +4 @ 26 SPM
1' at 2k pace +2 @ 28 SPM
1' at 2k pace +2 @ 30 SPM
12' rest
1' at 2k pace -2 @ 16 SPM
1' at 2k pace -2 @ 18 SPM
1' at 2k pace @ 20 SPM
1' at 2k pace @ 22 SPM
1' at 2k pace +2 @ 24 SPM
1' at 2k pace +2 @ 26 SPM
1' at 2k pace +4 @ 28 SPM
1' at 2k pace +4 @ 30 SPM

322. Get Tough

65-75 min.

Adv

8

TR

10' easy warm up
750m at 2k pace +6 @ 28 SPM, 3' rest
700m at 2k pace +6 @ 28 SPM, 3' rest
600m at 2k pace +4 @ 28 SPM, 3' rest
550m at 2k pace +4 @ 28 SPM, 3' rest
500m at 2k pace +2 @ 28 SPM, 3' rest
450m at 2k pace +2 @ 28 SPM, 3' rest
400m at 2k pace @ 28 SPM, 3' rest
350m at 2k pace -2 @ 28 SPM, 3' rest
300m at 2k pace -2 @ 28 SPM, 3' rest
250m at max @ 28 SPM, 3' rest
200m at max @ 28 SPM, 3' rest
150m at max @ 30 SPM, 3' rest
100m at max @ 32 SPM

323. Radar Island

52.5 min.

Adv

6

TR

10' easy warm up
2.5' at 2k pace -4 @ 28 SPM, 9' paddle pressure @ 22 SPM
2.5' at 2k pace -4 @ 28 SPM, 8' paddle pressure @ 22 SPM
2.5' at 2k pace -4 @ 30 SPM, 7' paddle pressure @ 22 SPM
2.5' at 2k pace -4 @ 30 SPM, 6' paddle pressure @ 22 SPM
2.5' at 2k pace -4 @ 32 SPM

ADVANCED

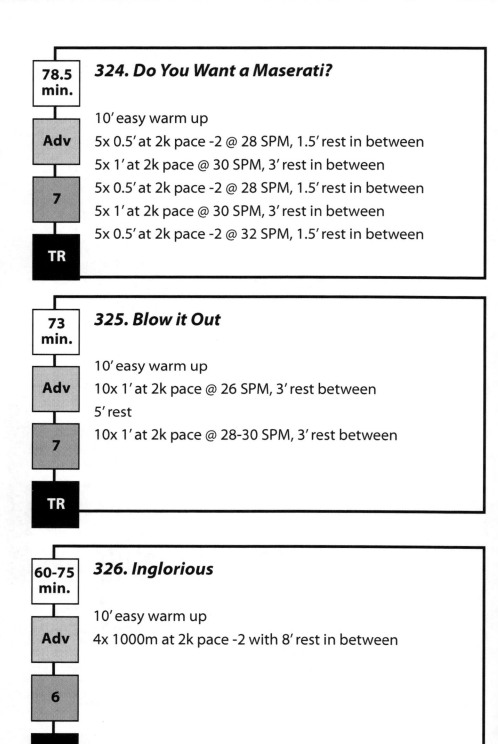

78.5 min.

Adv

7

TR

324. Do You Want a Maserati?

10' easy warm up
5x 0.5' at 2k pace -2 @ 28 SPM, 1.5' rest in between
5x 1' at 2k pace @ 30 SPM, 3' rest in between
5x 0.5' at 2k pace -2 @ 28 SPM, 1.5' rest in between
5x 1' at 2k pace @ 30 SPM, 3' rest in between
5x 0.5' at 2k pace -2 @ 32 SPM, 1.5' rest in between

73 min.

Adv

7

TR

325. Blow it Out

10' easy warm up
10x 1' at 2k pace @ 26 SPM, 3' rest between
5' rest
10x 1' at 2k pace @ 28-30 SPM, 3' rest between

60-75 min.

Adv

6

TR

326. Inglorious

10' easy warm up
4x 1000m at 2k pace -2 with 8' rest in between

327. Yesterday's Lunch

10' easy warm up

5x 750m at 2k pace -4 @ 28 SPM with 250m paddle in between

10' rest

5x 750m at 2k pace -4 @ 30 SPM with 250m paddle in between

65-80 min.

Adv

7

TR

328. Python

10' easy warm up

1000m at 2k pace -3 @ 24 SPM, equal time off

1000m at 2k pace -2 @ 26 SPM, equal time off

1000m at 2k pace -1 @ 28 SPM, equal time off

1000m at 2k pace @ 30 SPM, equal time off

1000m at 2k pace +1 @ 28 SPM, equal time off

1000m at 2k pace +2 @ 26 SPM, equal time off

1000m at 2k pace +3 @ 24 SPM

60-75 min.

Adv

9

TR

ADVANCED

329. Man Overboard

10' easy warm up

10x 3' at 2k pace +3 @ 28 SPM, 3' rest in between

67 min.

Adv

7

TR

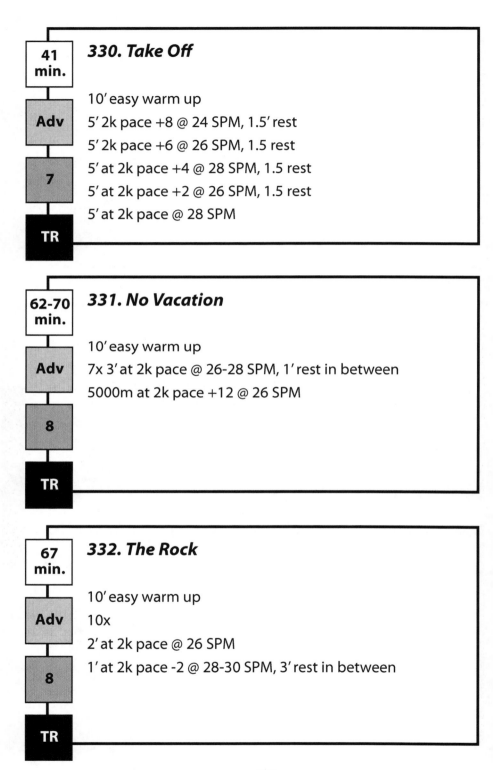

41 min.

Adv

7

TR

330. Take Off

10' easy warm up
5' 2k pace +8 @ 24 SPM, 1.5' rest
5' 2k pace +6 @ 26 SPM, 1.5 rest
5' at 2k pace +4 @ 28 SPM, 1.5 rest
5' at 2k pace +2 @ 26 SPM, 1.5 rest
5' at 2k pace @ 28 SPM

62-70 min.

Adv

8

TR

331. No Vacation

10' easy warm up
7x 3' at 2k pace @ 26-28 SPM, 1' rest in between
5000m at 2k pace +12 @ 26 SPM

67 min.

Adv

8

TR

332. The Rock

10' easy warm up
10x
2' at 2k pace @ 26 SPM
1' at 2k pace -2 @ 28-30 SPM, 3' rest in between

333. Africanized Bees

10' easy warm up

12x 500m at 2k pace -2 @ 34 SPM, 30 strokes paddle in between

58-65 min.

Adv

9

TR

334. The Captain

10' easy warm up

1500m at 2k pace +15 @ 28 SPM, 3' rest

9x 500m at 2k pace -2 @ 28 SPM, 1' rest in between

1500m at 2k pace +15 @ 28 SPM

55-65 min.

Adv

8

TR

ADVANCED

335. Tredegar's

10' easy warm up

24x 500m at 2k pace @ 28-32 SPM, 2' rest in between

105-115 min.

Adv

10

TR

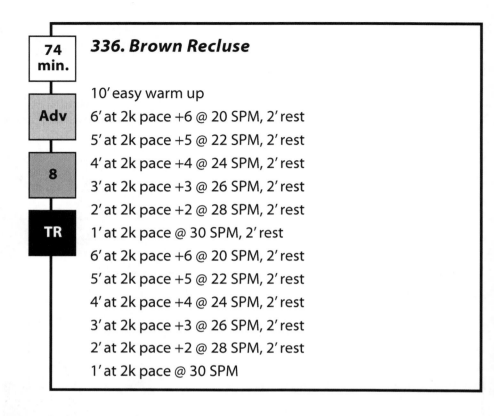

74 min.

Adv

8

TR

336. Brown Recluse

10' easy warm up
6' at 2k pace +6 @ 20 SPM, 2' rest
5' at 2k pace +5 @ 22 SPM, 2' rest
4' at 2k pace +4 @ 24 SPM, 2' rest
3' at 2k pace +3 @ 26 SPM, 2' rest
2' at 2k pace +2 @ 28 SPM, 2' rest
1' at 2k pace @ 30 SPM, 2' rest
6' at 2k pace +6 @ 20 SPM, 2' rest
5' at 2k pace +5 @ 22 SPM, 2' rest
4' at 2k pace +4 @ 24 SPM, 2' rest
3' at 2k pace +3 @ 26 SPM, 2' rest
2' at 2k pace +2 @ 28 SPM, 2' rest
1' at 2k pace @ 30 SPM

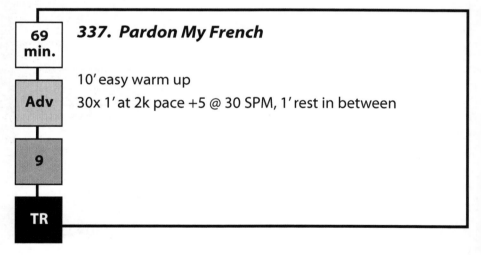

69 min.

Adv

9

TR

337. Pardon My French

10' easy warm up
30x 1' at 2k pace +5 @ 30 SPM, 1' rest in between

338. Yo Mamma's So Ugly

10' easy warm up
15x 500m at 2k -3 with 0.5' rest in between

40-55 min.

Adv

8

TR

339. Nutter Butter

10' easy warm up
1' at 2k pace +4 @ 25 SPM, 1' off
2' at 2k pace +6 @ 27 SPM, 2' off
3' at 2k pace +8 @ 29 SPM, 3' off
4' at 2k pace +6 @ 30 SPM, 4' off
5' at 2k pace +4 @ 32 SPM, 5' off
4' at 2k pace +2 @ 30 SPM, 4' off
3' at 2k @ 30 SPM, 3' off
2' at 2k -2 @ 32 SPM, 2' off
1' at 2k -4 @ max SPM

59 min.

Adv

8

TR

ADVANCED

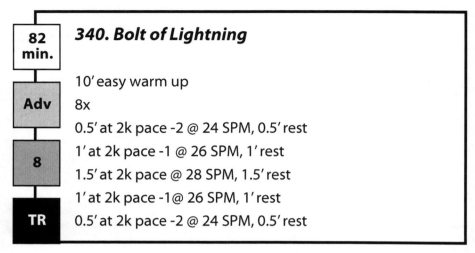

82 min.

Adv

8

TR

340. Bolt of Lightning

10' easy warm up

8x

0.5' at 2k pace -2 @ 24 SPM, 0.5' rest

1' at 2k pace -1 @ 26 SPM, 1' rest

1.5' at 2k pace @ 28 SPM, 1.5' rest

1' at 2k pace -1@ 26 SPM, 1' rest

0.5' at 2k pace -2 @ 24 SPM, 0.5' rest

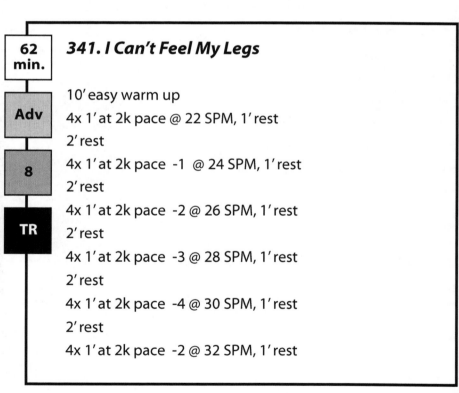

62 min.

Adv

8

TR

341. I Can't Feel My Legs

10' easy warm up

4x 1' at 2k pace @ 22 SPM, 1' rest

2' rest

4x 1' at 2k pace -1 @ 24 SPM, 1' rest

2' rest

4x 1' at 2k pace -2 @ 26 SPM, 1' rest

2' rest

4x 1' at 2k pace -3 @ 28 SPM, 1' rest

2' rest

4x 1' at 2k pace -4 @ 30 SPM, 1' rest

2' rest

4x 1' at 2k pace -2 @ 32 SPM, 1' rest

342. Vomit Comet

50-60 min.

Adv

10

TR

10' easy warm up
2000m at 2k pace +4
5' rest
2000m at 2k pace +8
5' rest
2000m at 2k pace + 6
5' rest
2000m at 2k pace +6

343. Duck, Duck, Goose

85-95 min.

Adv

9

TR

10' easy warm up
35x 150m on at 2k pace +4 @ 32 SPM, 150m paddle

ADVANCED

344. 100% Better

58-68 min.

Adv

9

TR

10' easy warm up
2000m at 2k pace +6 @ 28-32 SPM, 3' rest
1500m at 2k pace +4 @ 28-32 SPM, 3' rest
1250m at 2k pace +2 @ 28-32 SPM, 3' rest
1000m at 2k pace @ 28-32 SPM, 3' rest
750m at 2k pace @ 28-32 SPM, 3' rest
500m at 2k pace @ 28-32 SPM, 3' rest
250m at 2k pace @ 28-32 SPM

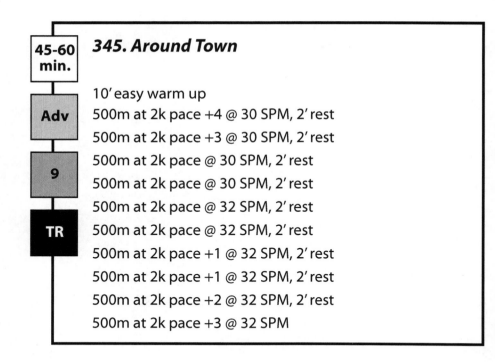

45-60 min.

Adv

9

TR

345. Around Town

10' easy warm up
500m at 2k pace +4 @ 30 SPM, 2' rest
500m at 2k pace +3 @ 30 SPM, 2' rest
500m at 2k pace @ 30 SPM, 2' rest
500m at 2k pace @ 30 SPM, 2' rest
500m at 2k pace @ 32 SPM, 2' rest
500m at 2k pace @ 32 SPM, 2' rest
500m at 2k pace +1 @ 32 SPM, 2' rest
500m at 2k pace +1 @ 32 SPM, 2' rest
500m at 2k pace +2 @ 32 SPM, 2' rest
500m at 2k pace +3 @ 32 SPM

346. Even Weirder Vibe

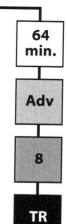

64 min.

Adv

8

TR

10' easy warm up
1' at 2k pace @ 16 SPM
1' at 2k pace @ 18 SPM
1' at 2k pace @ 20 SPM
1' at 2k pace @ 22 SPM
1' at 2k pace +2 @ 24 SPM
1' at 2k pace +2 @ 26 SPM
1' at 2k pace +2 @ 28 SPM
1' at 2k pace +2 @ 30 SPM
15' rest
1' at 2k pace +4 @ 16 SPM
1' at 2k pace +4 @ 18 SPM
1' at 2k pace +4 @ 20 SPM
1' at 2k pace +4 @ 22 SPM
1' at 2k pace +4 @ 24 SPM
1' at 2k pace +4 @ 26 SPM
1' at 2k pace +4 @ 28 SPM
1' at 2k pace +4 @ 30 SPM
15' rest
1' at 2k pace +6 @ 16 SPM
1' at 2k pace +6 @ 18 SPM
1' at 2k pace +6 @ 20 SPM
1' at 2k pace +6 @ 22 SPM
1' at 2k pace +6 @ 24 SPM
1' at 2k pace +6 @ 26 SPM
1' at 2k pace +6 @ 28 SPM
1' at 2k pace +6 @ 30 SPM

ADVANCED

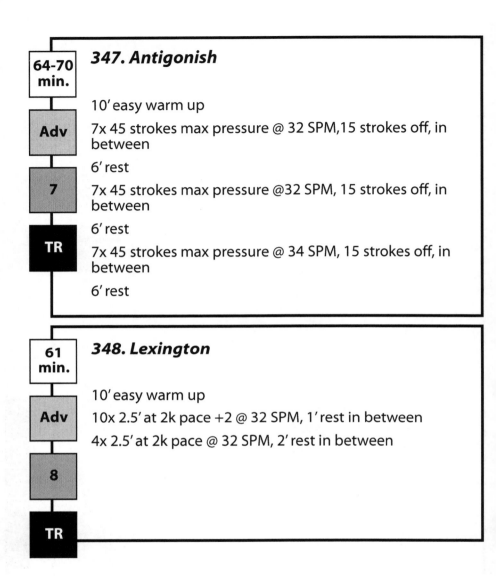

347. Antigonish

64-70 min.

Adv

7

TR

10' easy warm up

7x 45 strokes max pressure @ 32 SPM,15 strokes off, in between

6' rest

7x 45 strokes max pressure @32 SPM, 15 strokes off, in between

6' rest

7x 45 strokes max pressure @ 34 SPM, 15 strokes off, in between

6' rest

348. Lexington

61 min.

Adv

8

TR

10' easy warm up

10x 2.5' at 2k pace +2 @ 32 SPM, 1' rest in between

4x 2.5' at 2k pace @ 32 SPM, 2' rest in between

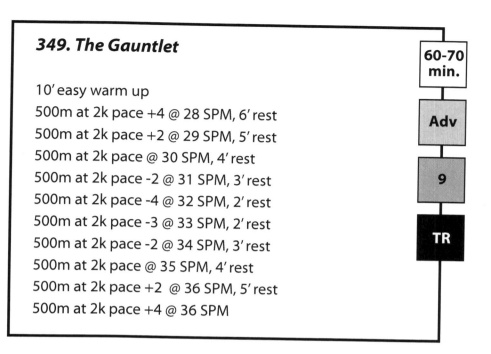

349. The Gauntlet

60-70 min.

Adv

9

TR

10' easy warm up
500m at 2k pace +4 @ 28 SPM, 6' rest
500m at 2k pace +2 @ 29 SPM, 5' rest
500m at 2k pace @ 30 SPM, 4' rest
500m at 2k pace -2 @ 31 SPM, 3' rest
500m at 2k pace -4 @ 32 SPM, 2' rest
500m at 2k pace -3 @ 33 SPM, 2' rest
500m at 2k pace -2 @ 34 SPM, 3' rest
500m at 2k pace @ 35 SPM, 4' rest
500m at 2k pace +2 @ 36 SPM, 5' rest
500m at 2k pace +4 @ 36 SPM

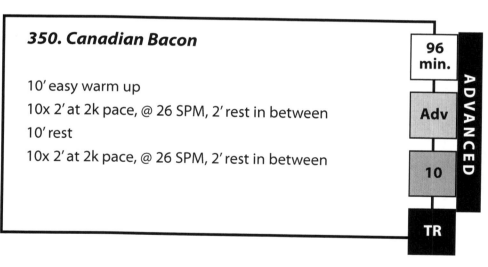

350. Canadian Bacon

96 min.

Adv

10

TR

ADVANCED

10' easy warm up
10x 2' at 2k pace, @ 26 SPM, 2' rest in between
10' rest
10x 2' at 2k pace, @ 26 SPM, 2' rest in between

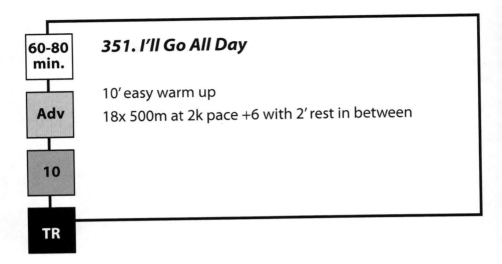

60-80 min.

Adv

10

TR

351. I'll Go All Day

10' easy warm up
18x 500m at 2k pace +6 with 2' rest in between

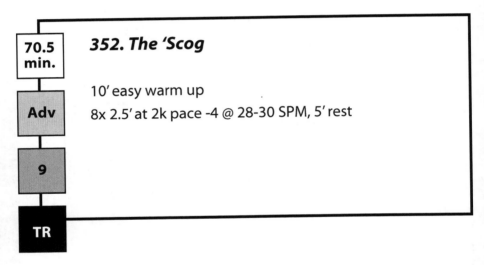

70.5 min.

Adv

9

TR

352. The 'Scog

10' easy warm up
8x 2.5' at 2k pace -4 @ 28-30 SPM, 5' rest

TEAM WORKOUTS

The team workouts in this book are designed for on-the-water rowing teams training in the off-season, and for group erg fitness classes. Team workouts can generally be done with only two people, but are geared toward a larger group, including groups with more people than ergs. These workouts are especially useful for coaches, classes and rowers who are running captain's practices. Almost all of the team workouts can be accomplished within the framework of a typical two-hour practice time.

We suggest incorporating weights, core exercises, and the body circuits included in this book into your team erg workouts, especially when you have more rowers than ergs. This gives people something to do instead of standing around waiting for ergs to open up and keeps everyone better engaged and focused.

Team Challenges

One of the ways we like to make land training, especially winter training, a bit more tolerable is to create a training challenge for the team. We have tried many different formats over the years, but it seems to work best when the team is broken up into evenly matched groups, and those groups compete against one another to win points over the course of the winter training period – typically 3-4 months. Some days should also be reserved as opportunities for rowers to earn individual points.

We've done team challenges with masters teams where everyone kicks in money and the winners share a pool. We have also run team challenges with juniors, college and masters groups where the winners are awarded prizes. Non-monetary prizes like making the coach wear a silly outfit, getting to pick the first workout back on the water or getting your name on a plaque at the boathouse also works as motivation. Generally, the more invested the team is, the better the prizes and the more effort the coach puts into making the game transparent and fair, the more fun the team has during winter training. Posting a leader board at the boathouse and making sure that workouts are fairly handicapped ensures that everybody, from the stars to the slowest on the team, has a chance to participate, win points for their groups and, ultimately make the team faster overall.

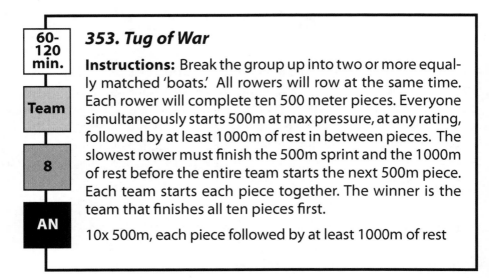

353. Tug of War

Instructions: Break the group up into two or more equally matched 'boats.' All rowers will row at the same time. Each rower will complete ten 500 meter pieces. Everyone simultaneously starts 500m at max pressure, at any rating, followed by at least 1000m of rest in between pieces. The slowest rower must finish the 500m sprint and the 1000m of rest before the entire team starts the next 500m piece. Each team starts each piece together. The winner is the team that finishes all ten pieces first.

10x 500m, each piece followed by at least 1000m of rest

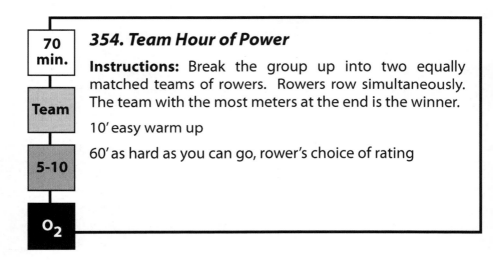

354. Team Hour of Power

Instructions: Break the group up into two equally matched teams of rowers. Rowers row simultaneously. The team with the most meters at the end is the winner.

10' easy warm up

60' as hard as you can go, rower's choice of rating

355. Movie Night

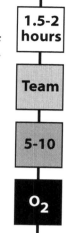

Instructions: As home indoor rowers know, one of the great distracters in aerobic training is watching TV or movies while working out. However, rowing teams generally don't seem to use it as much. We'll warn you that you'll need a good speaker system and will have to crank the volume up with lots of ergs going.

This one is pretty simple - find a movie you can tolerate. Break the group into two evenly divided teams based on 2k erg scores. Everyone starts together as the movie starts. Winner is the team with the most collective meters (or average meters per rower if the teams are unbalanced) at the final credits roll. We suggest any of the *Rocky* movies, but whatever works for your team.

Target pulling at 6k pace + 10 @ 24-26 SPM

1.5-2 hours

Team

5-10

O₂

356. Survival of the Fittest

Instructions: Break the group up into two or more evenly matched teams; (ideally) each team has the same number of rowers. Teams should not have more than 5 people on them, or it becomes too easy. Each team should have only one erg.

This is an ideal workout for a team with a limited number of ergs. The team can tackle a 20,000m piece collectively. Each rower has to row at least 2000m, and team members can go in any order and any number of 'turns' rowing. First team to finish the 20,000m piece is the winner.

20,000m at max pressure, any rating

50-75 min.

Team

7

AT

TEAM

Team

7-9

AT

357. The Tortoise and the Hare

Instructions: Pair the fastest and slowest rower together, the second fastest and second slowest and so on, so that everyone has a buddy. Do six pieces. Rest time starts when the slower rower finishes the piece. The faster rower should encourage the slower one as soon as he or she is done. Winner is the pair who has the lowest combined split, averaged over the six pieces.

6x 1500m at max pressure, with 5' rest in between, starting when the slower rower finishes

---

Team

7

AT

358. Rats in the Chimney

Instructions: Start with a 1k time trial, or organize your team based on previous 1k times. Line all of the ergs up such that rowers are sitting next to one another in a long line with the fastest team member at one end of the line and the slowest at the other end. Between each piece, reorganize rowers based on time. (We like to have them write down the times on a whiteboard between pieces). Winner is the rower who moved up the most seats during the workout. This one is good because even slower rowers can 'win' from the back. If you have significant difference between the fastest and slowest rowers on the team, consider splitting into a fast group and slow group, so that the faster rowers are not sitting around for too long in between pieces.

6x 1000m, 4' rest in between starting when the last rower finishes

359. Spin the Bottle

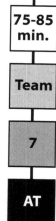

75-85 min.

Team

7

AT

Instructions: Organize rowers based on 2k erg times; arrange ergs in a large circle, up to 12 ergs, facing inward. If you have a bigger team, break into several erg circles. Rowers of similar 2k scores should be sitting near one another. Use a water bottle of some sort in the center of the circle. First rower will spin the water bottle to find out who they are challenging in the first 500m piece. The entire group starts the 500m piece together, although the only two rowers that are 'racing' are the rower who spins and the rower who the bottle lands on. At the end of the first 500m piece, the two rowers who were 'racing' compare to see which has the lowest negative split off their 2k time, and that person is the winner. The loser pushes his or her erg back one foot out of the circle, and the winner spins again. Only rowers in the inner circle are eligible to face off. Keep going as a group until there is one winner. The 'eliminated' rowers and 'non-racing' rowers will continue to do the rest of the pieces with the group at their 2k pace +6 split. This one is particularly good for mental training because it is impossible for rowers to tell who is winning the 'race' until it is over. This work out is also good for groups with big differences in speed because slower rowers can beat faster ones.

12x 500m pieces, with 5' rest in between

360. Out Kick Your Coverage

Instructions: This works best if rowers don't know what the game is until after they've done the first 1k. All rowers do a 1k time trial.

The idea is to go for a personal best 1k. After the 1k, break the group up into two or more evenly divided teams based on 1k times. Do another 1k for time – each rower earns points for his or her team. Seconds slower than the first 1k are added, and seconds faster than the first 1k are subtracted. Repeat as needed. The team with the lowest points total wins. This is best done in flights when teams have fewer ergs than rowers.

3-5x 1000m pieces with about 8' rest in between

361. The Stadium

Instructions: Break the group into evenly matched teams of 3 or 4 based on 2k times (the fastest two rowers in the group are teamed with the slowest two rowers, etc...). Each team gets one erg. Each team has to rotate through the pyramid.

It is up to the rowers to determine who goes in what order, but every team member has to do at least three complete pieces, one rower per piece, and no single rower can do two of the same length of piece (e.g. the same rower cannot pull both of the 250m pieces).

Pieces must be done in the order shown below, and optimal strategy is to perfect the handoff between rowers on and off the erg. The first team to finish wins.

10' warm up for all rowers

250m, 500m, 750m, 1000m, 1250m, 1500m, 1250m, 1000m, 750m, 500m, 250m at any rating

362. Be Honest

Instructions: Break the group into evenly matched teams of 4 based on 2k times (e.g. fastest two rowers in the group are teamed with the slowest two rowers, etc…). Teams get two ergs (at any time two rowers are rowing, and two are resting). The team with the most meters at the end wins. You can also do this with 2 rowers per team and one erg. No cheating on the off strokes is allowed.

10' easy warm up

10x 5' of 45 strokes full pressure, 15 off, followed by 5' of rest

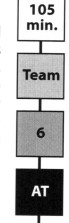

105 min.

Team

6

AT

363. Loch Ness Monster

Instructions: Break the team up into pairs, pairing the fastest rower with the slowest rower, the second fastest with the second slowest and so on. Each pair of rowers gets one erg. Set each erg to 13,000m. Rower A rests while Rower B is on the erg and vice versa. Rower A does a 3000m piece, then Rower B does a 3000m piece, then Rower A does a 2k and so on, switching back and forth.

You'll have to gage to make sure the transitions are quick and the meters are as close to accurate as possible. The fastest pair to complete the 13,000m wins. Rowers can row at any pressure and rate.

60-75 min.

Team

7

AT

10' easy warm up

Rower A 3000m

Rower B 3000m

Rower A 2000m

Rower B 2000m

Rower A 1000m

Rower B 1000m

Rower A 500m

Rower B 500m

TEAM

| 60 min. |
| Team |
| 2-10 |
| TR |

364. Bracketology

Instructions: Works best with groups of 8, 16, 32 or 64. Start with a 500m time trial, or organize your team based on previous 1k times. Seed everyone based on prior times and put into brackets, March Madness style, on a white board. Top seeds row against bottom seeds through the early rounds, regionals, semi-finals and final until there is one winner.

If you have an odd number of people, you can have rowers row twice or have a 'row in' to get into the bracket. This one is not particularly physically challenging for the majority of the team, but the fun quotient is high. Based on results, you can always re-seed and repeat. This is a great off-the-water practice for teams with more rowers than ergs.

500m pieces at max pressure, until you have a winner, 5' rest in between

Round of 64 takes about 60 minutes, if 'regions' start simultaneously

| 60-70 min. |
| Team |
| 8 |
| TR |

365. We Used to Be Friends

Instructions: Break the team up into pairs, pairing the fastest rower with the slowest rower, the second fastest with the second slowest and so on. Each pair of rowers gets one erg. Set the erg to 15,000m. Each rower rows 500m at a time, alternating rowers back and forth. While one rower is rowing, the other is resting.

You can make up significant time with good transitions. The pair that finishes the 15,000m first is the winner. This is great for team building and for teams with more rowers than ergs.

15x 500m pieces per rower

366. Raccoons in the Chimney

Instructions: Start with a 500m time trial, or organize your team based on previous 1k times. Line all of the ergs up such that rowers are sitting next to one another in a long line with the fastest team member at one end of the line and the slowest at the other end. Between each piece, reorganize rowers based on time. (We like to have them write down the times on a whiteboard between pieces).

Each piece is started simultaneously. Rest time starts ticking when the slowest rower has finished the work piece. Winner is the rower who moved up the most seats during the workout. This one is good because even slower rowers can 'win' from the back.

15x 500m, at least 2' rest in between

| 60 min. |
| Team |
| 8 |
| TR |

367. Four Chances

Instructions: Break the group up into teams of four rowers each. Teams should be evenly matched as possible. Each team gets one erg. Each rower will do a 2k at max pressure, one after the other, and then repeat, such that each rower will pull a 2k at max pressure twice with about 20-25 minutes of rest in between.

The winner is the first team to finish 16,000m. If you have three rowers on a team, they would only pull 12,000 meters total, teams of 5 would pull 20,000m total and so on.

16,000m total, each rower rows 2k at a time

| 50-80 min. |
| Team |
| 5-8 |
| TR |
| TEAM |

368. What Goes Up Must Come Down

Instructions: Break the team up into pairs, pairing the fastest rower with the slowest rower, the second fastest with the second slowest and so on. Each pair of rowers gets one erg. Set the erg to 16,200 meters.

Rower A rests while Rower B is on the erg and vice versa. Rower A goes up from 250m to 2k while Rower B goes down from 2k to 250m. The first sequence is Rower A pulls 250m, then switches, and Rower B gets on the erg and pulls 2000m. Then in the second sequence, Rower A pulls 500m, and Rower B pulls 1750m and so on, switching back and forth.

You'll have to gage to make sure the transitions are quick and the meters are as close to accurate as possible. The fastest pair to complete the 16,200m wins.

Rower A: 250m, 500m, 750m, 1000m, 1250m, 1500m, 1750m, 2000m, max pressure, any rate

Rower B: 2000m, 1750m, 1500, 1250m, 1000m, 750m, 500m, 250m, max pressure, any rate

369. Three is a Crowd

Instructions: Divide group into teams of three rowers. Stack the teams with the three best rowers on the first team, the next three fastest rowers in the second team and so on. Rowers will be individually competing against the other members of their team.

This one is great for teams with more rowers than ergs. Rower A pulls the first piece, followed by Rower B and then Rower C. Fastest aggregate time wins your group of three. This one is helpful to have a note pad or whiteboard to keep track of times.

250m, 500m, 750m, 1000m, 1500m, 2000m

370. Coach's Choice

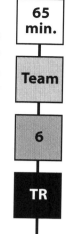

Instructions: Break the group up into two or more evenly matched teams. Ideally, each team has the same number of rowers. Ergs should be lined up in two rows facing each other, based on 2k times, with the fastest rowers on one end and the slowest at the other end.

The team with the most collective meters rowed at the end is the winner. It is helpful to have a whiteboard to keep track of meters and tabulate results.

10' easy warm up

8x 1.5' at max pressure, rower's choice of rating, 1' rest in between each

5' rest

8x 1' at max pressure, rower's choice of rating, 1' rest in between each

5' rest

8x 0.5' at max pressure, rower's choice of rating, 1' rest in between each

371. Extra Strength Deodorant

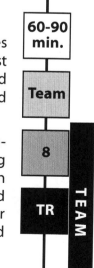

Instructions: Organize rowers based on 2k erg times and break into pairs. The fastest two rowers race against each other, rowers 3 and 4 race against each other and so on. Odd numbered rowers are on one team, and even numbered rowers are on the other team.

Set up the ergs facing each other with screens overlapping, so team A is facing one side, and Team B is facing the other side, but you can see the screen of the person you're racing against. First person who wins the head to head 'race' with his or her opponent wins a point for his or her team. Team with the most points at the end wins.

10' easy warm up

15,000m

32 min.

Team

7

TR

372. Frenemies

Instructions: Done in pairs, pair up the two strongest rowers, the next two and so on. One person's sprint time is the other person's rest time. Most meters wins the face-off and gets a point for the team. Team with the most points wins. Make sure you can see each other's screens.

Rower A-1' at full pressure any rating, Rower B resting

Rower B-1' at full pressure any rating, Rower A resting

Rower A-2' at full pressure any rating, Rower B resting

Rower B-2' at full pressure any rating, Rower A resting

Rower A-3' at full pressure any rating, Rower B resting

Rower B-3' at full pressure any rating, Rower A resting

Rower A-4' at full pressure any rating, Rower B resting

Rower B-4' at full pressure any rating, Rower A resting

Rower A-3' at full pressure any rating, Rower B resting

Rower B-3' at full pressure any rating, Rower A resting

Rower A-2' at full pressure any rating, Rower B resting

Rower B-2' at full pressure any rating, Rower A resting

Rower A-1' at full pressure any rating, Rower B resting

Rower B-1' at full pressure any rating, Rower A resting

373. Target on Your Back

Instructions: Split the team into two or more equally matched 'boats' of an equal number of people, (preferably 4 or 8 people) and line the ergs up into rows of 'boats.' All team members erg at the same time, following and matching, stroke for stroke, the person sitting in 'stroke' erg.

During rest pieces everyone moves back one erg, and the person at the back moves up to the 'stroke' erg. The winning boat is the 'stroke' with the best average split for the last piece.

2' at full pressure @ 18 SPM, 2' at full pressure @ 20 SPM, 4' rest

2' at full pressure @ 20 SPM, 2' at full pressure @ 22 SPM, 4' rest

2' at full pressure @ 22 SPM, 2' at full pressure @ 24 SPM, 4' rest

2' at full pressure @ 24 SPM, 2' at full pressure @ 26 SPM, 4' rest

2' at full pressure @ 26 SPM, 2' at full pressure @ 28 SPM, 4' rest

1' at full pressure @ 28 SPM, 1' at full pressure @ 30 SPM, 2' rest

1' at full pressure @ 30 SPM, 1' at full pressure @ 32 SPM, 2' rest

0.5' at full pressure @ 32 SPM, 0.5' at full pressure @ 34 SPM

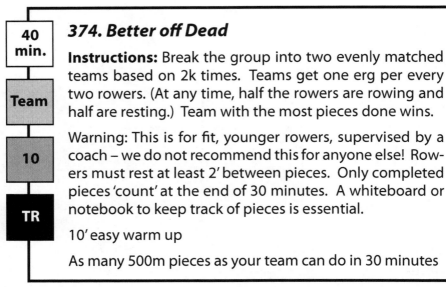

374. Better off Dead

40 min.

Team

10

TR

Instructions: Break the group into two evenly matched teams based on 2k times. Teams get one erg per every two rowers. (At any time, half the rowers are rowing and half are resting.) Team with the most pieces done wins.

Warning: This is for fit, younger rowers, supervised by a coach – we do not recommend this for anyone else! Rowers must rest at least 2' between pieces. Only completed pieces 'count' at the end of 30 minutes. A whiteboard or notebook to keep track of pieces is essential.

10' easy warm up

As many 500m pieces as your team can do in 30 minutes

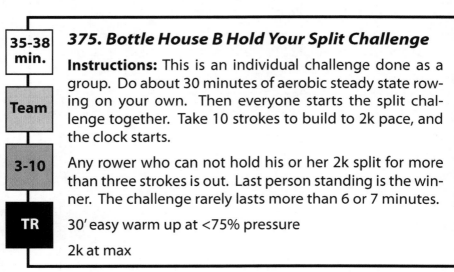

375. Bottle House B Hold Your Split Challenge

35-38 min.

Team

3-10

TR

Instructions: This is an individual challenge done as a group. Do about 30 minutes of aerobic steady state rowing on your own. Then everyone starts the split challenge together. Take 10 strokes to build to 2k pace, and the clock starts.

Any rower who can not hold his or her 2k split for more than three strokes is out. Last person standing is the winner. The challenge rarely lasts more than 6 or 7 minutes.

30' easy warm up at <75% pressure

2k at max

376. Fight Club Hold Your Split Challenge

35-38 min.

Team

3-10

TR

Instructions: This is a variation on the Bottle House B and is also an individual challenge done as a group. Do about 30 minutes of aerobic steady state rowing on your own. Then everyone starts the split challenge together. Take 10 strokes to build to 2k pace, and the clock starts. Any rower who falls below his or her 2k split for more than three strokes is out.

After the first minute of the challenge, the pace drops to 2k -1. At the second minute, the pace drops to 2k pace -2 and so on. Any rower who can not hold his or her target split for more than three strokes is out. Last person standing is the winner. The challenge rarely lasts more than 4 or 5 minutes.

30' easy warm up at <75% pressure

1' at 2k pace, 1' at 2k pace -1, 1' at 2k pace -2, 1' at 2k pace -3, 1' at 2k pace -4, 1' at 2k pace -5, 1' at 2k pace -6, etc... (you'll never get that far!)

TEAM

377. Minor League Erging

Instructions: Variations on erg baseball abound, but we like the basic version best. Break your team into evenly matched groups based on average 2k split time. Each rower's individual 2k time will be used to calculate points.

Points are scored for each 'inning' using the chart below which will involve adding up individual scores at the end. The 'game' is run on 6 minute centers. In other words, every six minutes, everyone on the team starts a new 500m piece together. Do nine innings or 9 x 500m total. The team with the most points at the end wins it. Points are assessed for each inning as follows:

2k pace -4 or better	Grand Slam	5
2k pace -3 or better	Home Run	4
2k pace -2 to 2k pace -3	Triple Play	3
2k pace -1 to 2k pace -2	Double Play	2
2k pace to 2k pace -1	Single	1
2k pace to 2k pace +1	Foul Ball	0
2k split +1 to 2k pace +2	Out	-1
2k split +2 to 2k pace +3	Double (for the other team)	-2
2k split +3 or over	Unforced Error	-3

378. Erg Baseball – Midwestern Version

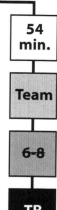

54 min.

Team

6-8

TR

Instructions: Break your group into evenly matched teams based on average 2k split time. Line the ergs up in two lines, head to head, with the fastest two rowers facing one another and so on down the line.

Each rower's individual 2k time will be used to calculate points. Everybody rows 9 x 500m pieces, starting together, on 6 minute centers. Your first 500m piece (or 'inning') starts with your slowest pair. Have them go head to head. Only that pair, the rowers 'up to bat,' can score points for the team for that piece.

For the second 500m piece, move to your next slowest pair and so on, until all of the pieces are done. Everyone not 'up to bat' should be at 2k split. Anyone caught sandbagging (taking it easy) when they are not 'up to bat' could face a suspension, and the other team automatically wins that inning. Points are assessed as follows:

2k pace -4 or better	Grand Slam	5
2k pace -3 or better	Home Run	4
2k pace -2 to 2k pace -3	Triple Play	3
2k pace -1 to 2k pace -2	Double Play	2
2k pace to 2k pace -1	Single	1
2k pace to 2k pace +1	Foul Ball	0
2k split +1 to 2k pace +2	Out	-1
2k split +2 to 2k pace +3	Double (for the other team)	-2
2k split +3 or over	Unforced Error	-3

TEAM

BODY CIRCUIT EXERCISES

BODY CIRCUITS FOR INDOOR ROWING

Body circuit exercises are a perfect addition to your erg workouts, whether you're rowing on your own or training for on-the-water rowing with a team. These exercises are good for all levels and will help elevate your indoor rowing workouts by improving balance, flexibility and strength. We include more than 20 of the best rowing-specific body circuit exercises that can be done without anything more than boat straps and chairs from around the boathouse. Weights, yoga mats and fitness balls are luxury additions if you have them, but are not really necessary. You can also add in whatever types of weights you have on hand, from sand bags and ancient pieces of boathouse detritus to actual weight lifting equipment.

All of these exercises can be incorporated into your active rest between erg pieces. These are typically done in sets of 10x, 20x or 50x or repeatedly for 1-2 minutes. You'll want to adapt to your specific needs, workout plan and abilities.

We'll also mention that if your body cannot handle significant impact, you should refrain from the exercises that involve jumping or lifting off of the ground.

1. Burpies

This classic rowing exercise, often inflicted by rowing coaches as punishment, works your entire body.

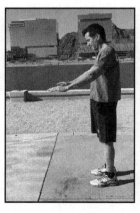 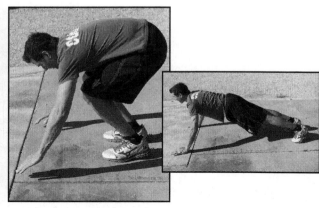

A. Start by standing with feet shoulder width apart.

B. Bend your knees and kick your legs out, dropping down to a push up position (Remember to keep your rear end down).

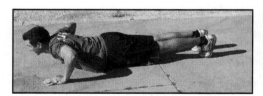 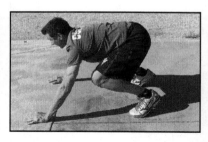

C. Drop into a push up until your chest touches the ground, then push back up.

D. Jump back into a squat position, and

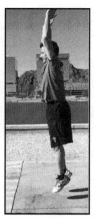

E. Finally jump up, getting your feet off of the ground.

2. Air Squats

Air squats focus on the legs and require no additional equipment.

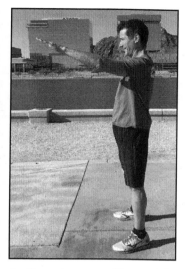

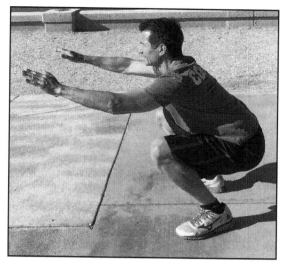

A. Start by standing with feet shoulder width apart and arms extended.

B. Deeply bend your knees, dropping down below the height you'd be sitting in a chair, continuing to keep arms extended.

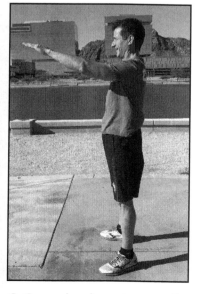

C. Come back up to standing position with arms still extended.

3. Planks

Planks are ideal for building core strength. Typically, planks are held in position for a minute or more, but if you're just starting out, try a plank position for ten seconds, building up until you can hold for a minute. We show both forward plank and side plank position here.

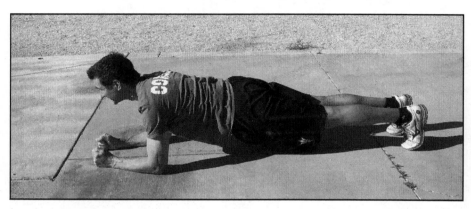

A. In forward plank position, you'll balance your weight on both fore-arms and both feet simultaneously, focusing on keeping your rear end down and your back flat and straight.

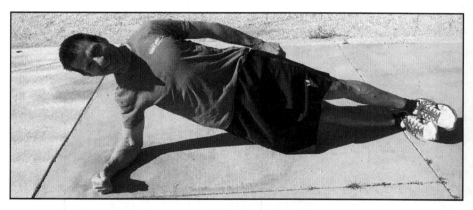

B. In side plank position, you'll balance your weight on one forearm and the side of one foot, focusing on keeping your body in a nice diagonal line to the ground, and not breaking at the waist. After you do side plank on one side, do the other side.

4. Pushups

Pushups are a classic gym exercise that you are undoubtedly familiar with. Here we show both regular pushups and modified pushups for those with less upper body strength. In both, you'll want arms shoulder width apart with hands even on the floor and your weight balanced evenly on both feet (regular) or on both knees (modified).

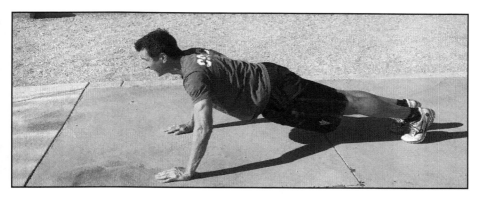

A. Start a regular push up with arms straight and back flat, focusing on keeping your rear end down.

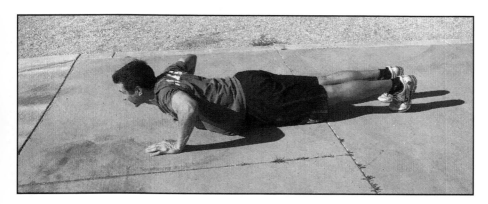

B. With a regular pushup, focus on keeping the body flat as you bend your arms, trying to get your elbows fully bent. Then go back to starting position.

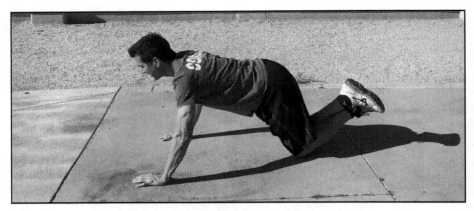

C. Start a modified pushup with arms straight and back flat, focusing on pushing down evenly on both sides of the body.

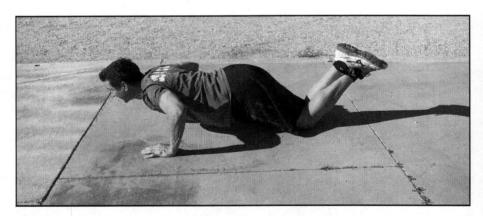

D. With a modified pushup, drop the arms as low as you can, trying to keep your rear end down and getting the elbows as bent as possible. Then go back to starting position.

5. Crunches

Crunches target the core, specifically the abdominal muscles. You can do these on an exercise ball or mat to make it more comfortable. You want to make sure that you're using the abdominal muscles to lift your torso off of the ground, not pulling up or straining your neck.

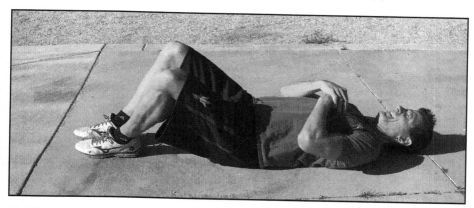

A. Make sure your knees are shoulder width apart with weight even on both feet and cross your arms across your chest.

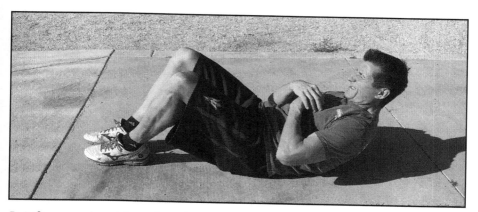

B. Lift your shoulders, head and upper torso off of the floor. Then go back to starting position.

6. Butterfly Sit ups

Butterfly sit ups work the core muscles, especially the abdominal muscles. You can use a mat to make the exercise more comfortable. Put the bottoms of your feet together, spreading your knees out enough to allow your arms between them.

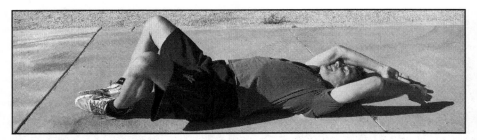

A. Lay on your back with the bottoms of your feet together and your arms above your head, grasping at the wrists.

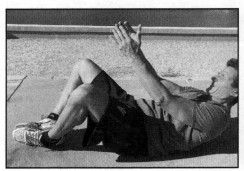 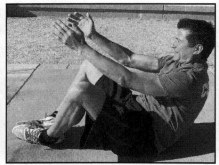

B. With your arms extended, bring your arms forward and lift your shoulders and torso up off the floor.

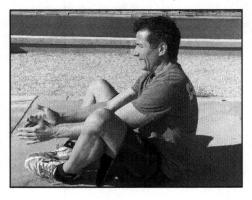

C. Move into sitting position with your arms outstretched between your legs. Reverse back to starting position.

7. L Sits

L sits are another solid core exercise for rowing and work the abdominal muscles, back and shoulders. Make sure you have two sturdy well-balanced chairs. You can also use bleachers, weight benches, boxes or other types of furniture.

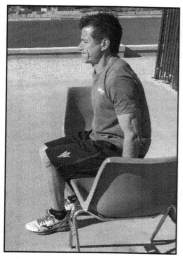
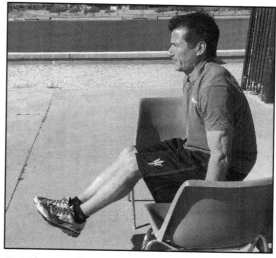

A. Place two chairs about shoulder width apart, and move into a seated position with weight evenly balanced on both arms.

B. Lift your legs up off of the ground, balancing on your arms only and pushing your legs away from the body.

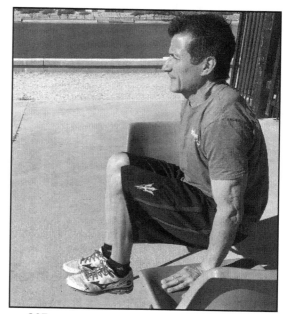

C. Bring the legs back toward the chest. Repeat, moving your legs away from and back toward the body, or return to your feet on the ground.

8. Wall Walkers

Wall walkers require a little balance and a wall or (less ideally) someone to hold your feet. This is a full body exercise and uses all sorts of muscles. Wearing shoes with a good grip is essential to avoid falling on your face.

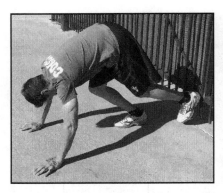

A. Facing away from the wall, place your hands on the floor at shoulder width apart and the soles of your shoes on the wall.

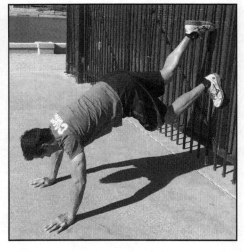

B. Walk your feet up the wall, walking your arms closer to the wall as you go.

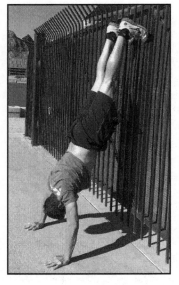

C. Go up to a handstand position with legs and arms fully outstretched. Walk back down the wall to starting position.

9. Mountain Climbers

Mountain climbers are another rowing staple exercise that works your core muscles.

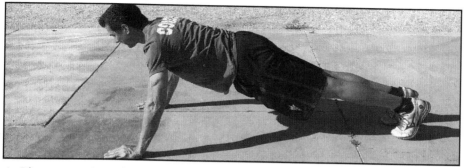

A. Place your hands shoulder width apart on the floor, balancing your weight evenly on hands and feet.

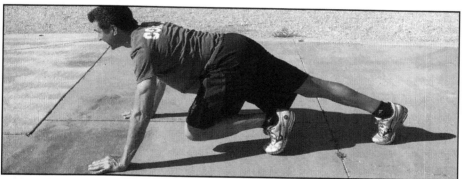

B. In a jumping motion , bend your left knee under you, focusing on keeping the back straight. Then kick the left leg back out to starting position.

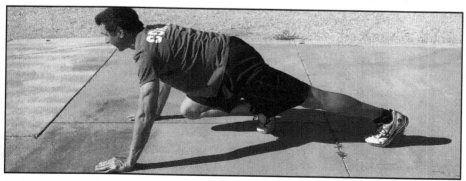

C. Repeat on the right side. In a jumping motion, bend your right knee under you, focusing on keeping the back straight. Then kick the right leg back out to starting position. Repeat, alternating legs.

10. Step ups

Step ups are used to strengthen leg muscles and rower reflexes. This exercise can be done on a set of stairs, bleachers, stadiums or on a wooden box or low wall. Ideally the box is about 9-18 inches tall.

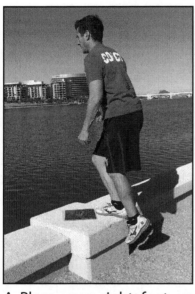 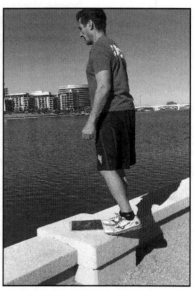

A. Place your right foot up onto the step. This foot will stay in place.

B. Bring your left foot up onto the step.

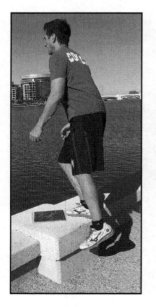 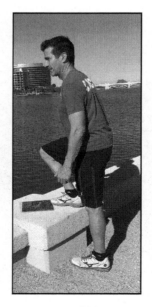

C. Bring your left foot back to the floor, keeping your right foot up on the step. Repeat, bringing the left foot up and down in rapid succession for a set number of repetitions or until your left leg fatigues. Then switch sides.

11. Lunges

Lunges are another great exercise for building leg muscles used in rowing. Lunges can be done without any equipment whatsoever, or you can do them with weights.

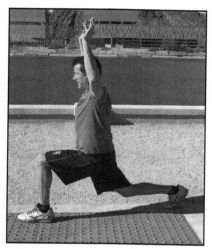
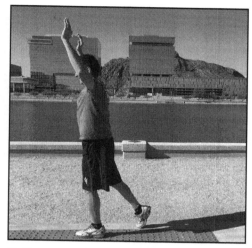

A. Lower into lunge position with your left leg bent at a 90-degree angle and your right foot stretched behind onto the ball of your right foot. Arms should be raised above head in a smooth sweeping motion.

B. Keeping both hands outstretched above your head, return to standing.

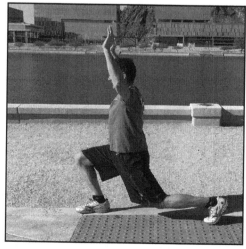

C. Lower into lunge position with your right leg bent at a 90-degree angle and your left foot stretched behind onto the ball of your left foot. Arms should stay raised above head. Then return to standing and repeat, alternating sides.

12. Jumping Jacks

This schoolyard staple has stood the test of time for a good reason - jumping jacks are a superb full body exercise. What's more, they are well suited to cross training for rowing. You can add resistance to jumping jacks with light arm weights or resistance bands.

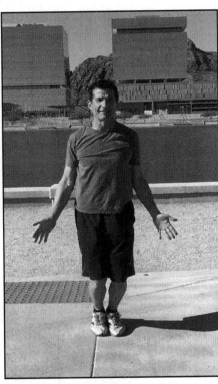 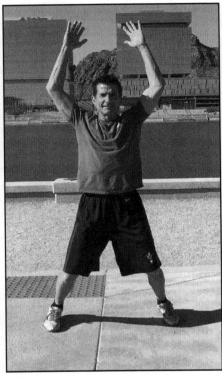

A. Stand with feet shoulder width apart and arms at the sides.

B. While jumping, kick your legs out to the sides and simultaneously bring your hands above your head in a smooth sweeping motion. Jumping again, return to feet together and arms by the sides. Repeat.

13. Chair Dips

As the name implies, chair dips require two sturdy chairs. If you don't have chairs handy, you can use bleachers, weight benches, boxes or other types of furniture. This exercise is focused on the upper body, especially the bicep and tricep muscles. Place two chairs about two feet apart. Arms should be outstretched to your sides about six inches, and your weight should be evenly balanced on both hands.

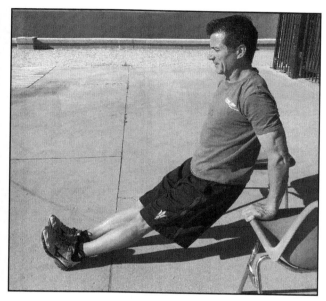

A. Start with your weight evenly balanced on your heels and your hands, bending slightly from the waist.

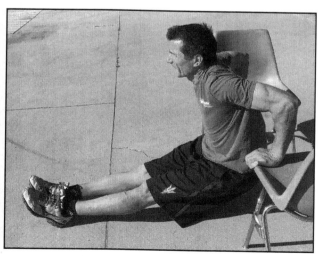

B. Bending from the waist, drop as low as you can go by bending your elbows. Return to starting position, and repeat as necessary.

14. Russian Twists

Russian twists are the answer when regular crunches become too easy or boring. This core exercise can be made more comfortable with the addition of a yoga mat. Start on your back with your weight balanced on your rear end, with legs up off the ground, knees slightly bent and elbows at a 90-degree angle.

A. From the waist, twist your arms to your left side, focusing on engaging your abdominal muscles to stabilize your torso.

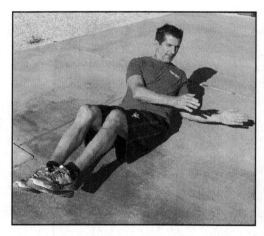

B. Keeping the legs in the same position, twist to the center, bringing your arms upright.

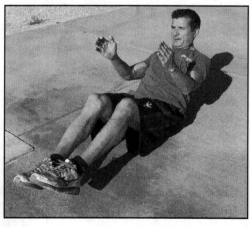

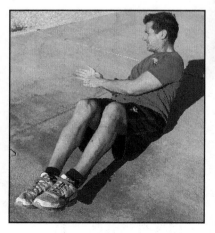

C. Keeping the legs in the same position, twist to your right, bringing your arms to the right. Repeat, alternating sides.

15. Calf Hops

Calf hops are a simple lower body focused workout that is ideal for rowing - the explosive power is the same motion you use in the pushing off your foot stretchers.

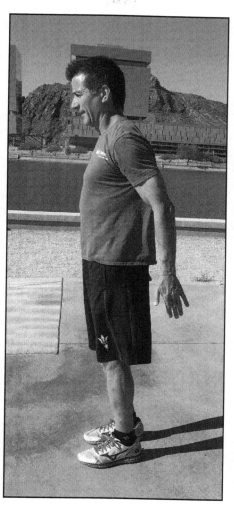
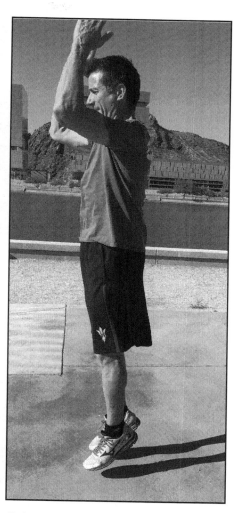

A. Stand with feet shoulder width apart, arms outstretched and slightly behind you.

B. In a sweeping motion, bring the arms up above your head, and jump up off the ground, pointing your toes as you go. Repeat.

16. Nordic Hamstring Curls

With a name like Nordic hamstring curls, you know it has to be a good exercise for rowers. This lower body focused exercise requires something to hook your legs under (such as bleachers, a fence, bar or bench), or a workout buddy to hold your feet. A mat for your knees makes it less painful but is not 100% necessary.

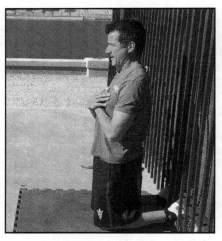 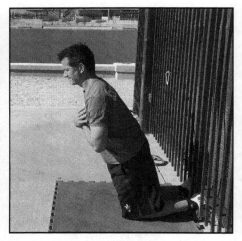

A. On your knees, hook your heels against the bar, and cross your arms across your chest.

B. Keeping your back as straight as possible, lean forward with your arms crossed across your chest until you get near the ground.

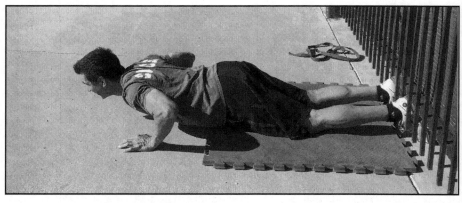

C. As you near the ground, put your arms down into a push up position.

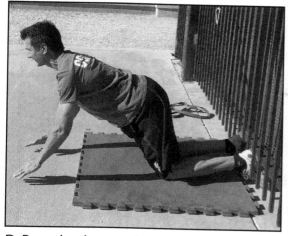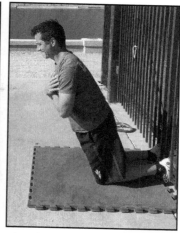

D. Press back up, using your legs to lift your body back up and crossing your arms.

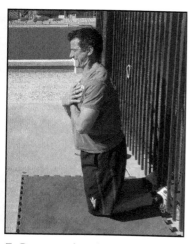

E. Return back to upright position. Repeat.

17. Super Heroes

The super hero is a basic core exercise for rowers. A yoga mat will make it slightly more enjoyable. It seems so easy, but it will make your abdominal muscles burn like crazy.

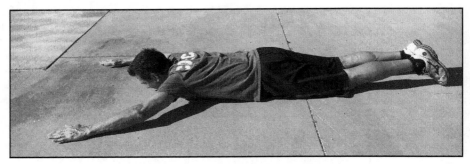

A. Lay on your belly with arms outstretched in front and legs behind.

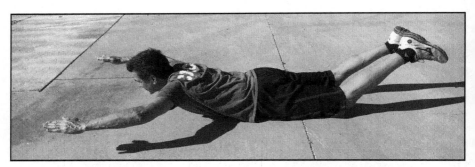

B. Simultaneously lift your arms and legs off of the floor. Hold until the point of fatigue. Repeat.

18. Body Rows

This upper body exercise uses your body weight for resistance. Body rows require a 12-foot boat strap, which is pretty common in most boathouses. If you don't have one on hand, you can use resistance bands or a length of rope. You'll loop the strap around something sturdy – a wall, fence, bleachers or something else that will not fall when you pull on it. A yoga mat will also make your knees feel better but is not 100% necessary.

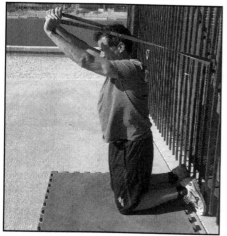 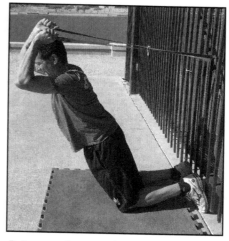

A. On your knees, with your legs shoulder width apart, body straight, and arms straight and outstretched in front of you, loop your hands against the strap.

B. Lean forward, keeping your body as straight as possible, and bend your elbows to a 90-degree angle, holding the strap in your hands. Return to starting position and repeat.

19. Arm Curls

If you want buff arms fast, arm curls are a great choice. Arm curls require a 12-foot boat strap, which is pretty common in most boathouses. If you don't have one on hand, you can use resistance bands or a length of rope. You'll loop the strap around something sturdy - a wall, fence, bleachers or something else that will not fall when you pull on it.

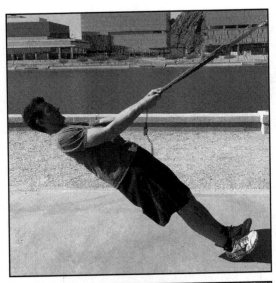

A. Lean back with your body completely straight, body weight balanced on your heels and arms outstretched straight in front of you holding the strap.

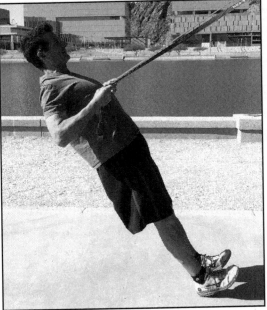

B. Holding the strap, keeping your weight on your heels and your body completely straight, bend your elbows to a 90-degree angle, pulling yourself up. Return to starting position and repeat.

20. Tricep Extensions

As you might expect, tricep extensions are upper body focused. Tricep extensions require a 12-foot boat strap, which is pretty common in most boathouses. If you don't have one on hand, you can use resistance bands or a length of rope. You'll loop the strap around something sturdy – a wall, fence, bleachers or something else that will not fall when you pull on it. You can also substitute arm weights for the strap.

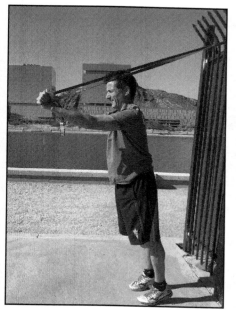 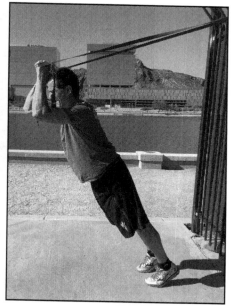

A. Stand with your feet shoulder width apart and with your weight on the balls of your feet. Your arms should be extended straight in front of you holding onto the strap.

B. Lean forward, keeping your body completely straight and your weight on the balls of your feet by bending your elbows to a 90-degree angle. Return to starting position, focusing on the resistance against your triceps.

21. Wall Ball

Wall ball exercises work lots of different muscle groups and are good for general flexibility. You ideally want to use a weighted ball, but you can substitute with anything really – playground ball, tennis ball, sand bag, backpack filled with your rowing gear – whatever works.

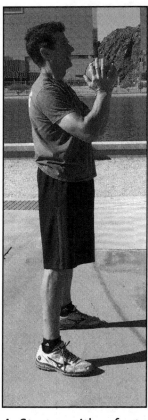 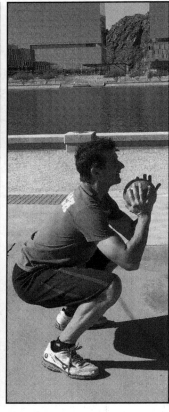 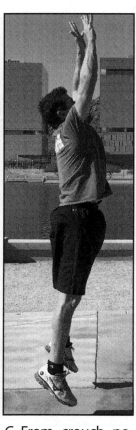

A. Start with feet shoulder width apart and arms at a 90 degree angle holding the ball near your head.

B. Keeping the arms bent at 90 degrees and the ball up by your face, bend your knees into a crouch position.

C. From crouch position, jump up off the ground, bringing your hands above your head, and project the ball against the wall. The object is to catch the ball as it bounces back off the wall. Repeat.

Made in the USA
Columbia, SC
20 November 2018